ACUPUNCTURE

OF

ACUPOINT

combinations

quick lookups

Editor

Guo Changqing

Published by

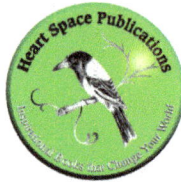

Heart Space Publications
PO Box 1085
Daylesford
Victoria
3460
Australia
Tel +61 450260348
www.heartspacebooks.com
pat@heartspacebooks.com

ISBN 978-0-6489215-5-4

Contents

Chapter 3 Trunk Combination Points   29

Chapter 5 Systemic Combination Points   111

Abstract

The book is compiled and edited by senior specialists and professors of the School of Acupuncture, Moxibustion, and Massage of Beijing University of Chinese Medicine.

Combination acupoints are two or more acupoints with the same or similar effects. The acupoints in the acupoint group cooperate with each other and play a therapeutic role in coordination, which can improve the curative effect. This book focuses on describing the main treatment, standard orientation, acupoint selection techniques of each combination acupoint, acupoint anatomy, acupuncture.

Acupoints can be accurately selected according to the images, which is convenient for clinical application of combined acupoints.

The book is applicable to both teachers and students of TCM colleges (in China and abroad, foreign students, and amateurs), universities, as well as professional clinical practitioners.

This is one of four books in the **Quick Reference Handbooks of Chinese Medicine series**

Testimonial

Excellent book illustrated with detailed and accurate deplaning pictures. It is a good guidance for both leaners and professionals.

Shen Weihong

Australian registered Chinese medical doctor and acupuncturist, council member of Federation of Chinese Medicine & Acupuncture Societies of Australia Ltd.

Foreword

Acupuncture and moxibustion is an important part of traditional Chinese medicine. Since ancient times, acupuncture and moxibustion therapy has been known to be simple, practical and effective. Attention has been paid by doctors throughtout the dynasties to relieve the suffering of the broad masses of the people and ensure their health.

Acupuncture and moxibustion treatment is based on acupoints, and all treatment measurments are through acupoints. Therefore, acupoint science plays an important role in acupuncture and moxibustion. Combination points are an important part of acupoint science and consists of two parts with the same or similar functions. In the acupoint group composed of two or more acupoints, the acupoints in the acupoint group cooperate with each other to play a therapeutic role.

Acupuncture, and or moxibustion, as single points may not alleviate symptoms. However, often, two or more acupoints are needed. In long-term and extensive clinical practice, doctors constantly sum up their experience and realise that some acupoints can be used together to synergize and improve the curative effect, some conventional acupoint groups were formed. In this way, the concept of combined acupoints is gradually formed.

This book is the result of intensive research of some common acupoint groups from ancient texts of acupuncture and moxibustion, according to head and neck. The order of combined acupoints of the trunk, limbs, and the entire body is discussed in turn. We hope that the publication of this book can promote the clinical application of combined acupoints.

Editor Guo Changqing
April, 2019

CHAPTER 1

Methods of Locating Combination Points

Section 1
Finger-length Measurement

Finger measurement is a method of standard measurement, for the location of the acupuncture point, since the fingers are in proportion with the other parts of the body – that the length and width of the patient's fingers are taken.

1. Four-Finger Measurement

The width of the four fingers (index, middle, ring and little) placed together, taken at the level of the dorsal crease of the proximal interphalangeal joint of the middle finger measures 3 cun. Cun is the term for the measurement relative to the patient (see images below). This method is always used to locate the points in the abdomen, back and lower limbs.

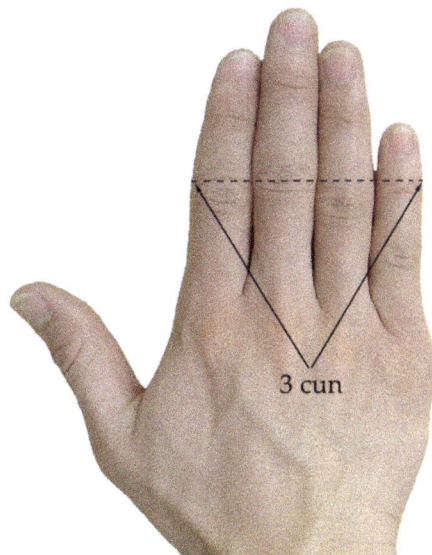

2. Thumb Measurement

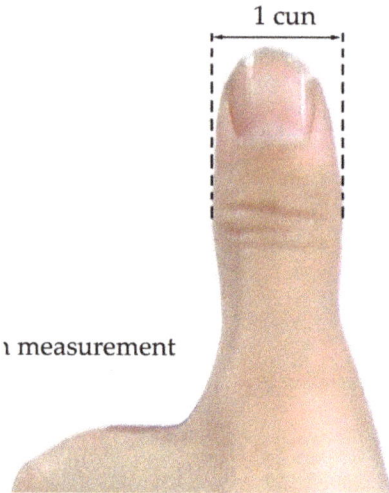

1 cun

ı measurement

Place the thumb straight. The width of the interphalangeal joint of the patient's thumb is 1 cun.

3. Middle Finger Measurement

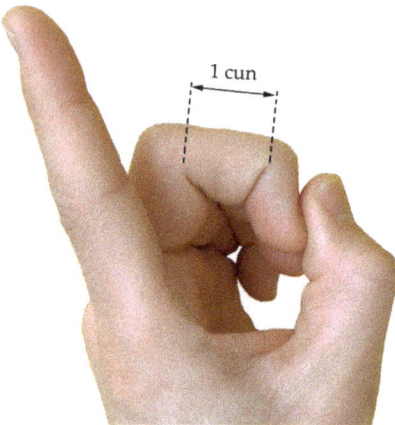

1 cun

When the patient's middle finger is flexed, the index finger is straight, and the end of the middle finger against the belly of the thumb, forming a ring. The width between the two medial ends of the creases of the interphalangeal joints is 1 cun. This method is suitable for limbs and transverse measurement of the dorsal.

Section 2
Bone-Length Measurement

The commonly used modern method of orientation of "bony degree" is based on Ling Shu (superior pivot), and in the long-term medical practice after modification and supplement, see the table below for details.

Standard for Bone-Length Measurement

Body Part	Area between two points on the body	Length in cun
Head	From the midpoint of the anterior hairline to the midpoint of the posterior hairline	12 cun

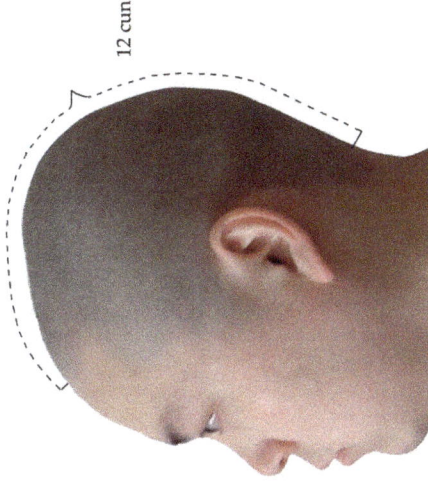

12 cun

Head	Between the corners of the forehead ST 8.	9 cun	
Head	Between the two mastoid processes	9 cun	
Chest and Abdomen	From the suprasternal fossa to the sternocostal angle	9 cun	
	From the sternocostal angle to the center of the umbilicus	8 cun	
	From the center of the umbilicus to the upper of symphysis pubis	5 cun	
	Between the two nipples	8 cun	

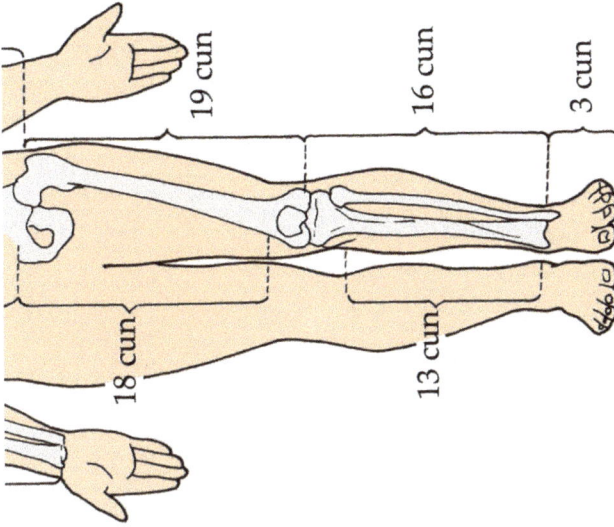

Lateral side of the trunk	From the tip of the axillary fossa to the tip of the 11th rib.	12 cun	
	From the tip of the 11th rib to the prominence of the great trochanter	9 cun	
Upper Limbs	From the end of the axillary fold to the transverse cubital crease	9 cun	
	From the transverse cubital crease to the transverse wrist crease	12 cun	
Lower Limbs	From the level of the border of symphysis pubis to the medial epicondyle of the femur	18 cun	
	From the lower border of the medial condyle of tibia to the tip of medial malleolus	13 cun	
	From the prominence of the great trochanter to the middle of patella	19 cun	
	From the center of patella to the tip of lateral malleolus	16 cun	
	From the tip of lateral malleolus to the sole.	3 cun	

.

CHAPTER 2

Head and Neck Combination Points

1. EX-HN 1, DU-24, GB-13 — Calms the spirit and benefits the brain, benefits the head and eyes

Indications	Headache, insomnia and epilepsy, manic psychosis, dizziness, poor memory.

EX-HN 1 — SìShénCōng

Position	A group of 4 points, at the vertex, 1 cun posterior, anterior and lateral to DU 20.
Acupoint Selection Skills	The point is located in the sitting or supine position, at the vertex, 1 cun posterior, anterior and lateral to DU 20.
Regional Anatomy	The needle passes through the subcutaneous tissues and reaches the loose connective tissue beneath aponeurosis and periost.
Acupuncture	Insert the needle subcutaneously towards DU 20, or insert 0.5~0.8 cun deep and stimulate until there is a sore and distending sensation in the local area.

DU-24 — ShénTíng

Position	On the head, 1 cun superior to the midpoint of the anterior hairline.
Acupoint Selection Skills	The point is located in the sitting or supine position, 0.5 cun superior to the midpoint of the anterior hairline.
Regional Anatomy	The needle passes through the skin and subcutis, penetrates galeaaponeurotica and reaches the deeper layer.
Acupuncture	Insert the needle subcutaneously 0.3~0.5 cun deep and stimulate until there is a heavy and distending sensation in the local area.

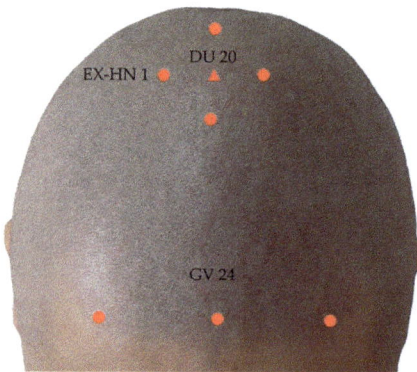

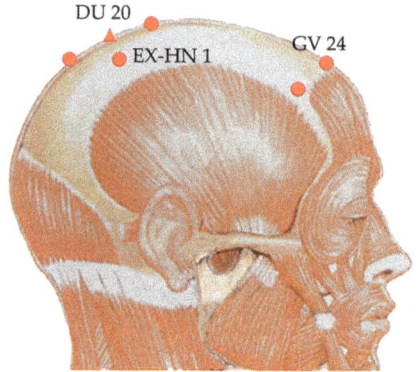

GB-13 — BěnShén

Position	On the head, 0.5 cun within the anterior hairline of the forehead, 3 cun lateral to DU 24.
Acupoint Selection Skills	The point is located in the sitting or supine position, 0.5 cun within the anterior hairline of the forehead, 3 cun lateral to DU 24, at the junction of the medial 2/3 and the lateral 1/3 of the line connecting DU 24 to ST 8.
Regional Anatomy	The needle passes through the subcutaneous tissues and penetrates the connective tissue beneath galeaaponeurotica.
Acupuncture	Insert the needle subcutaneously 0.5~0.8 cun deep and stimulate until there is a sore and numbing sensation in the local area

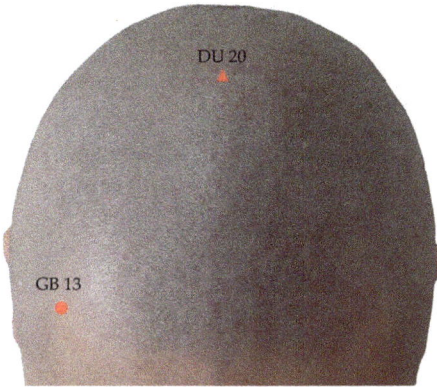

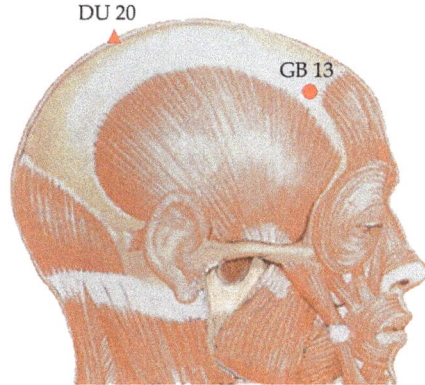

2. GB-5, GB-4 — Benefits the ears, expels wind and activates the channel

Indications	Headache, tinnitus and deafness, dizziness.

GB-5 — XuánLú

Position	In the hairline of the temporal region, at the midpoint of the arc between ST 8 and GB 7.
Acupoint Selection Skills	The point is located in the sitting or lateral position by first locating ST 8 and GB 7. GB 5 is located in the center of the arc between the two points.
Regional Anatomy	The needle passes through the subcutaneous tissues and penetrates the temporal fascia and m. temporalis.
Acupuncture	Insert the needle subcutaneously 0.5~0.8 cun deep and stimulate until there is a sore and numbing sensation in the local area.

GB-4 — HànYàn

Position	In the hairline of the temporal region, at the junction of the upper 1/4 and the lower 3/4 of the arc connecting ST 8 and GB 7.
Acupoint Selection Skills	The point is located in the sitting or lateral position, by first locating ST 8 and GB 7. GB 5 is in the center of the arc between these two points and GB 4 is in the middle of ST 8 and GB 5, in the upper 1/4 and the lower 3/4 of the arc connecting ST 8 and GB 7. By chewing food, where it moves, is the point.
Regional Anatomy	The needle passes through the subcutaneous tissues and penetrates the temporal fascia and m. temporalis.
Acupuncture	Insert the needle subcutaneously 0.3~0.5 cun deep and stimulate until there is a sore and numbing sensation in the local area.

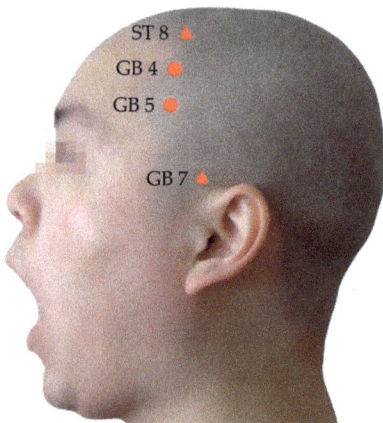

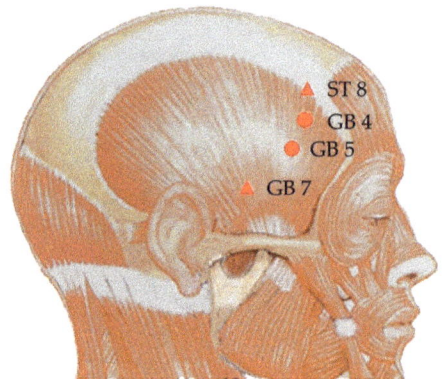

3. GB-2, SJ-17 — Benefits the ears, activates the channel and calms the spirit.

Indications	Headache, deviation of the eye and mouth, tinnitus and deafness, dizziness.

GB-2 — TīngHuì

Position	On the face, anterior to the intertragic notch, on the posterior border of the condyloid process of the mandible, in the depression when the mouth is open.
Acupoint Selection Skills	The point is located in the sitting position with an open mouth, in the depression anterior to the intertragic notch, on the posterior border of the condyloid process of the mandible.
Regional Anatomy	The needle passes through the subcutaneous tissues and penetrates the tissue near the parotid gland.
Acupuncture	Insert the needle perpendicularly 0.5~1.0 cun deep and stimulate until there is a sore and numbing sensation in the local area.

SJ-17 — YìFēng

Position	Posterior to the lobule of the ear, in the depression between the mastoid process and the angle of the mandible.
Acupoint Selection Skills	The point is located in the sitting by folding the lobule of the ear, in the depression anterior to the mastoid process.
Regional Anatomy	The needle passes through the skin and subcutaneous fascia, penetrates the masseteric fascia of parotid, and finally reaches the retromandibular prognathism of parotid.
Acupuncture	Insert the needle perpendicularly 0.8~1.2 cun deep and stimulate until there is a sore and numbing sensation in the local area radiating to the anterior parts of tongue and face.

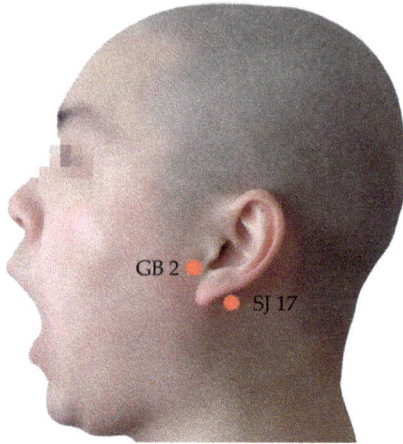

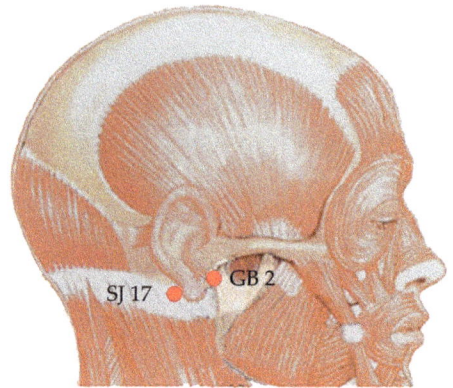

4. ST-8, GB-15 — Benefits the head and eyes, calms the spirit

Indications	Headache, redness, swelling and pain of the eye, tinnitus and deafness and unconscious.

ST-8 — TóuWéi

Position	On the head, 0.5 cun inside the anterior hairline above the temples and 4.5 cun from the midline.
Acupoint Selection Skills	The point is located on the head, on the line connecting GB 15 and DU 24, 4.5 cun lateral to DU 24, 0.5 cun within the hairline.
Regional Anatomy	The needle passes through the subcutaneous tissues and enters the m. temporalis.
Acupuncture	Insert the needle subcutaneously towards the back of the head 0.5~1.0 cun deep until there is a sore or distending sensation in the local area.

GB-15 — TóuLínQì

Position	On the forehead, directly above GB 14, 0.5 cun within the anterior hairline.
Acupoint Selection Skills	The point is located in the sitting or supine position, 0.5 cun within the anterior hairline, at the midpoint of the line connecting DU 24 to ST 8.
Regional Anatomy	The needle passes through the subcutaneous tissues and penetrates the connective tissue beneath galeaaponeurotica.
Acupuncture	Insert the needle subcutaneously 0.5~0.8 cun deep and stimulate until there is a sore and numbing sensation in the local area.

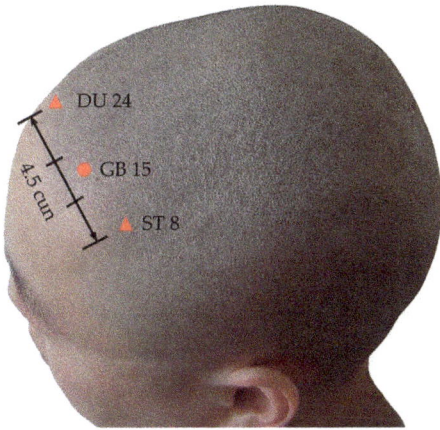

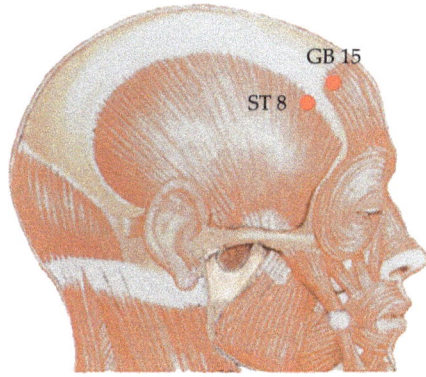

5. DU-17, GB-19 — Benefits the head and eyes, calms spirit

Indications	Headache, epilepsy, fright, neck stiffness, dizziness, ataxia and mental retardation.

DU-17 — NāoHù

Position	On the head, in the depression superior to the external occipital protuberance.
Acupoint Selection Skills	On the head, 2.5 cun superior to the midpoint of the posterior hairline, 1.5 cun anterior to DU 16, in the depression superior to the external occipital protuberance.
Regional Anatomy	The needle passes through the subcutaneous tissues and m. occipitofrontalis and penetrates the connective tissue beneath aponeurosis.
Acupuncture	Insert the needle subcutaneously 0.5~0.8 cun deep and stimulate until there is a sore and distending sensation in the local area.

GB-19 — NăoKōng

Position	On the head, on the lateral aspect of the superior border of the external occipital protubearance, directly above GB 20.
Acupoint Selection Skills	The point is located in the sitting or prone position, directly above GB 20, 2.25 cun lateral to the midline of the head, at the level with DU 17.
Regional Anatomy	The needle passes through the subcutaneous tissues and penetrates the m. occipitofrontalis.
Acupuncture	Insert the needle subcutaneously 0.5~0.8 cun deep and stimulate until there is a sore and numbing sensation in the local area radiating to the posterior parts of the head.

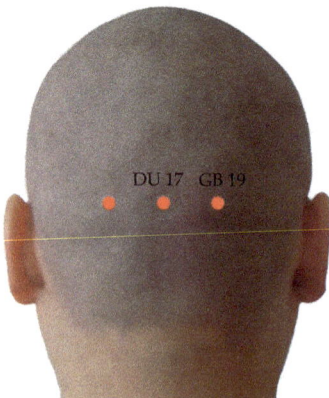

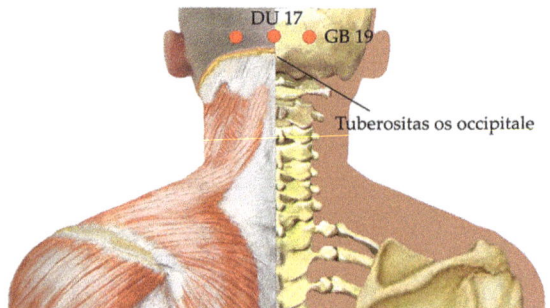

DU 17 GB 19

DU 17 GB 19

Tuberositas os occipitale

6. EX-HN 5, EX-HN 3 — Calms spirit, expels wind and clears heat

Indications	Trigeminal neuralgia, insomnia, epilepsy, dizziness, epistaxis, redness, swelling and pain of the eye.

EX-HN 5 — TàiYáng

Position	In the depression about one finger breadth posterior to the midpoint between the lateral end of the eyebrow and the outer canthus.
Acupoint Selection Skills	The point is located in the sitting or supine position, in the depression about one finger breadth posterior to the midpoint between the lateral end of the eyebrow and the outer canthus.
Regional Anatomy	The needle passes through the subcutaneous tissues and penetrates the m. temporalis near the superficial temporal artery and vein.
Acupuncture	① Insert the needle perpendicularly 0.3~0.5 cun deep and stimulate until there is a sore and distending sensation in the local area. ② Insert the needle backwards subcutaneously towards GB 8 1.0~2.0 cun deep and stimulate until there is a sore and distending sensation in the local area radiating to the temporal side.

EX-HN 3 — YìnTáng

Position	On the face, midway between the medial ends of the two eyebrows.
Acupoint Selection Skills	The point is located in the sitting or supine position, at the midpoint of the medial ends of the two eyebrows.
Regional Anatomy	The needle passes through the subcutaneous tissues and penetrates the m. procerus and m. corrugator supercilii and reaches frontal periost.
Acupuncture	Lift and squeeze the skin, insert the needle subcutaneously downwards 0.3~0.5 cun deep and stimulate until there is a sore and distending sensation in the local area.

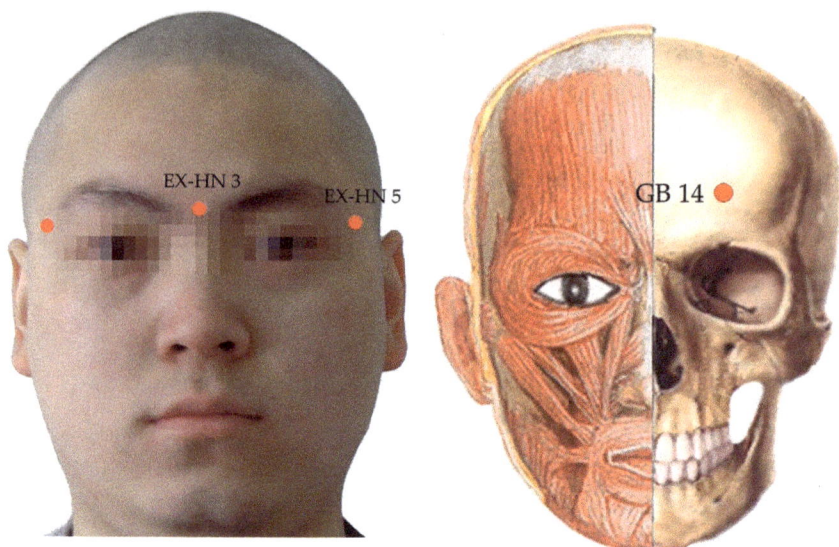

EX-HN 3
EX-HN 5
GB 14

7. BL-1, ST-1, EX-HN 7 — Expels wind and clears heat, improving vision and dissipates phlegm

Indications	Redness, swelling and pain of the eye, lacrimation, itching of the inner canthus, blurred vision and myopia, glaucoma, night blindness, optic nerve inflammation, strabismus.

BL-1 — JīngMíng

Position	On the face, in the depression superior to the inner canthus.
Acupoint Selection Skills	The point is located in the sitting position while looking upward or in the supine position, 0.1 cun superior to the inner canthus.
Regional Anatomy	The needle passes through the subcutaneous tissues and penetrates the m.rectusmedialis.
Acupuncture	Insert the needle slowly perpendicularly 0.3~0.5 cun deep while the eyes are closed by pushing the eyeball outwardly without lifting, thrusting, twisting and rotating the needle.

ST-1 — ChéngQì

Position	On the face, directly inferiorto the pupil while looking forward, between the eyeball and the infraorbital margin.
Acupoint Selection Skills	The point is located in the sitting or supine position while looking forward, in the depression between the eyeball and the infraorbital margin.
Regional Anatomy	The needle passes through the subcutaneous tissues and m. tarsalis inferior and enters the m. oblique inferior and m. rectus inferior.
Acupuncture	Push the eyeball upwards and hold with the left thumb. Insert the needle slowly perpendicularly 0.5~0.8 cun deep along the infraorbital ridge. Avoid manipulating the needle with large amplitude.

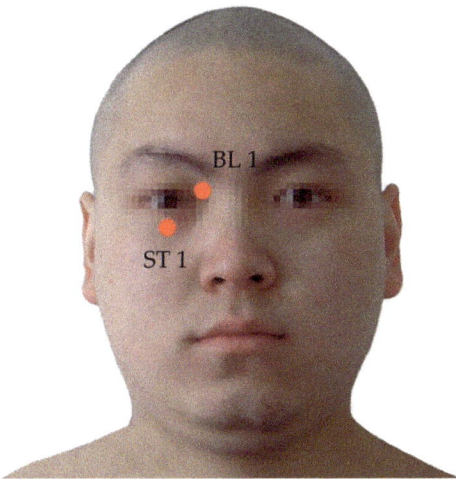

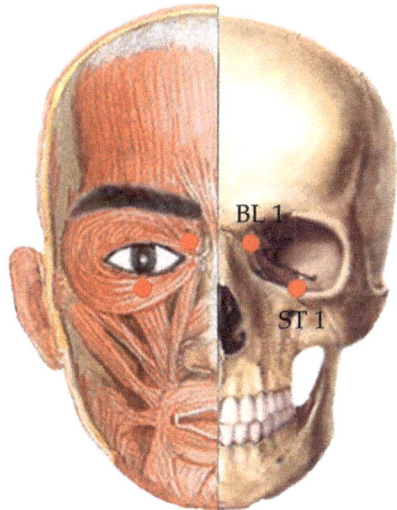

EX-HN 7 — QiúHòu

Position	At the junction of the lateral 1/4 and the medial 3/4 of the infraorbital margin.
Acupoint Selection Skills	The point is located in the sitting or supine position when the eyes are closed, at the junction of the lateral 1/4 and the medial 3/4 of the infraorbital margin.
Regional Anatomy	The needle passes through the subcutaneous tissues and penetrates the m. orbicularis oculi, m. tarsalis inferior, m. oblique inferior, corpus adiposumorbitae and reaches m. rectus inferior.
Acupuncture	Push the eyeball upwards gently, inserting the needle perpendicularly 0.3-0.5 cun deep slowly without lifting, thrusting, twisting and rotating the needle.

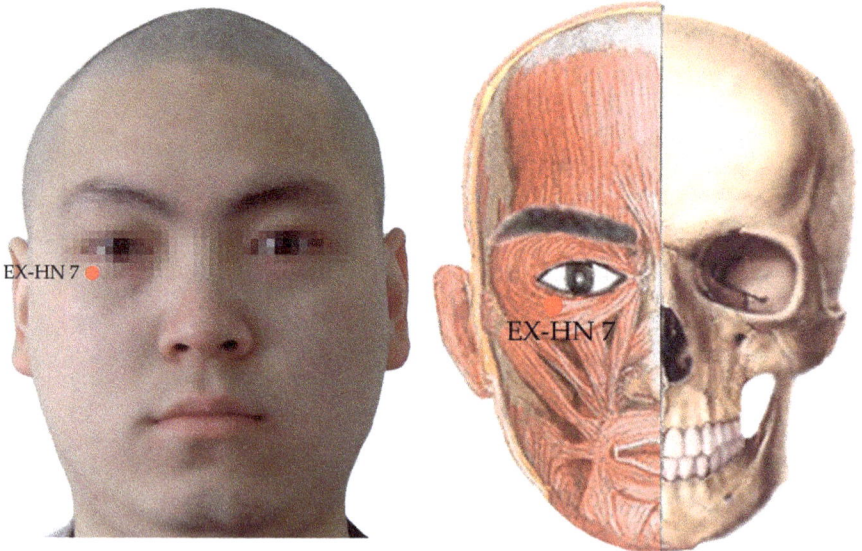

8. ST-4, ST-6, ST-7, GB-14 — Expels wind and alleviates pain, activates the channel and activates collaterals

(collateral: refers to the route of the Chi flowing through people's body. Collateral refers to the branches, not the main flowing route).

Indications	At the junction of the lateral 1/4 and the medial 3/4 of the infraorbital margin.

ST-4 — DìCāng

Position	On the face, directly inferior to ST 3 at the level with the corner of the mouth.
Acupoint Selection Skills	The point is located in the sitting or supine position while looking forward, the point is directly inferior to the pupil at the level of the corner of the mouth.
Regional Anatomy	The needle passes through the subcutaneous tissues, penetrates between m. risorius and m. buccinator and enters the masseter.
Acupuncture	Insert the needle subcutaneously 1.0~2.5 cun deep towards ST 6 and stimulate until there is a sore and numbing sensation in the local area.

ST-6 — JiáChē

Position	On the cheek, in the depression one finger-breadth anterior and superior to the corner of the mandible.
Acupoint Selection Skills	The point is located in the sitting or recumbent position on the prominence of the masseter when the teeth are clenched, which becomes a depression when the masseter m. is relaxed.
Regional Anatomy	The needle passes through the subcutaneous tissues, penetrates the deep fascia of masseter and enters the masseter.
Acupuncture	Insert the needle subcutaneously towards ST 4 1.0~2.0 cun deep and stimulate until there is a sore and numbing sensation in the local area.

ST-7 — XiàGuān

Position	In the depression between the zygomatic arch and mandibular notch in front of the ear.
Acupoint Selection Skills	The point is located in the sitting or recumbent position, on the inferior border of the zygomatic arch, anterior to the condyloid process of the mandible.
Regional Anatomy	The needle passes through the posterior aspect of the parotid, penetrates the m. temporalis, and enters infratemporal fossa.
Acupuncture	Insert the needle perpendicularly 1.0~1.5 cun deep and stimulate until there is a sore and numbing sensation in the local area.

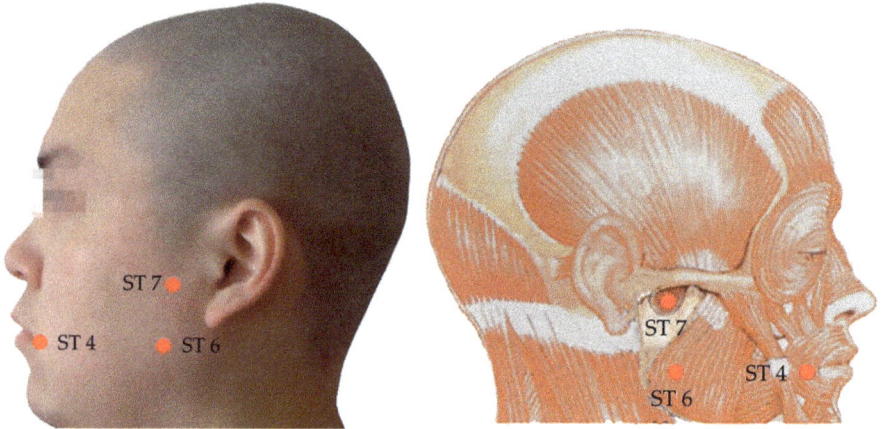

GB-14 — YángBái

Position	On the forehead, directly above the pupil, 1 cun superior to the eyebrow.
Acupoint Selection Skills	The point is located in the sitting or supine position, 1 cun superior to the eyebrow, directly above the pupil when looking forward.
Regional Anatomy	The needle passes through the subcutaneous tissues and penetrates the connective tissue beneath galeaaponeurotica.
Acupuncture	Insert the needle subcutaneously 0.5~0.8 cun deep and stimulate until there is a sore and numbing sensation in the local area.

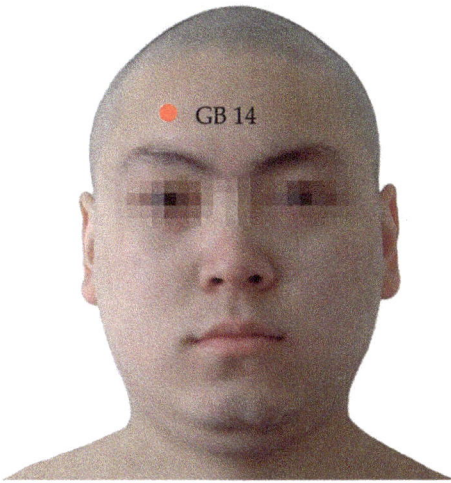

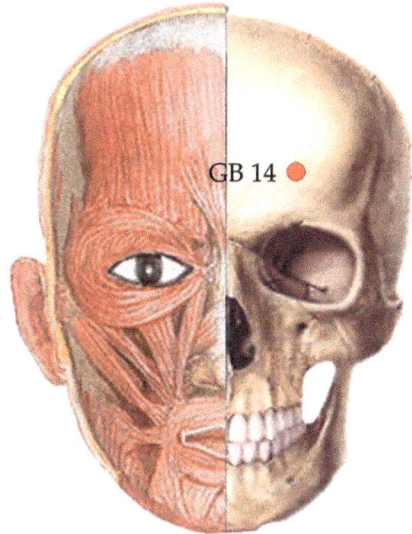

9. RN-23, DU-15 — Clears heart and benefits the throat, benefits the tongue and treats muteness

Indications	Deaf and mute syndrome, sudden loss of the voice, swelling and pain of the tongue, aphtha of the mouth and tongue.

RN-23 — LiánQuán

Position	On the neck, on the anterior midline, above the Adam's Apple, in the depression above the upper border of the hyoid bone.
Acupoint Selection Skills	The point is located in the sitting or supine position, above the Adam's Apple, in the depression above the upper border of the hyoid bone.
Regional Anatomy	The needle passes through subcutis and penetrates the thyroid gland, hyoid bone and median ligament.
Acupuncture	Insert the needle perpendicularly 0.5~0.8 cun deep then withdraw the needle to the superficial level and stimulate by reinserting obliquely right and left until there is a sore and distending sensation in the local area.

DU-15 Y — Mén

Position	On the back of the neck, superior to the spinous process of the second cervical vertebra, on the posterior midline.
Acupoint Selection Skills	The point is located in the sitting position when the head bends forwards slightly, 0.5 cun superior to the posterior hairline.
Regional Anatomy	The needle passes through the subcutaneous tissues and penetrates the nuchal ligament and interarcuate ligament.
Acupuncture	Insert the needle perpendicularly 0.5~0.8 cun deep and stimulate until there is a sore and numbing sensation in the local area. Avoid deep insertion to prevent injury to the spinal cord.

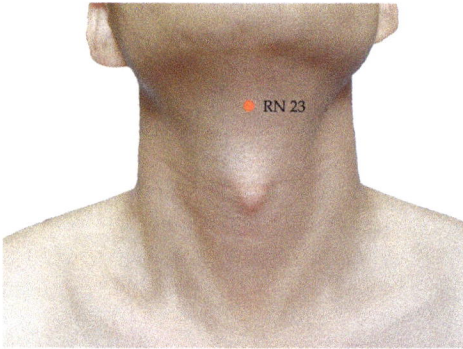

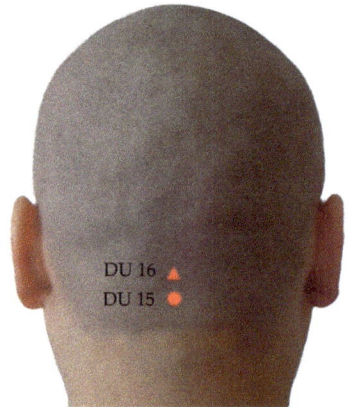

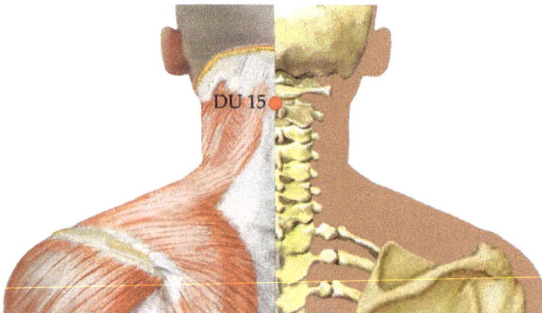

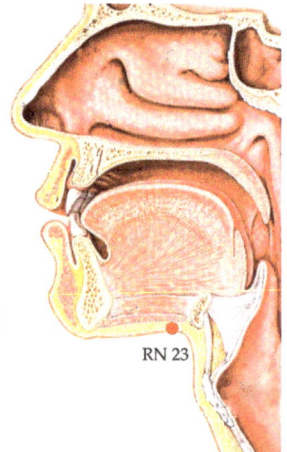

10. GB-20, BL-10, DU-14 — Expels wind and strengthens exterior, activates channel

Indications	Headache and fever, cough and asthma, neck stiffness, pain of the shoulder and back, rubella, epilepsy and infantile convulsions, redness, swelling and pain of the eye.

GB-20 — FēngChí

Position	On the nape, below the occipital bone, in the depression between m. sternocleidomastoideus and m. trapezius.
Acupoint Selection Skills	The point is located in the sitting or prone position, on the nape, in the depression lateral and inferior to the occipital, between m. sternocleidomastoideus and m. trapezius.
Regional Anatomy	The needle passes through the subcutaneous tissues and penetrates the m. rectus capitis posterior major.
Acupuncture	Insert the needle downwards and inwards obliquely 0.5~1.5 cun deep and stimulate until there is a sore and numbing sensation in the local area.

BL-10 — TiānZhù

Position	On the neck, in the depression on the lateral border of m. trapezius, superior to the spinous process of the second cervical vertebra.
Acupoint Selection Skills	The point is located in the sitting position with the head bent forward or in the prone position, 1.3 cun lateral to DU 15, lateral to m. trapezius.
Regional Anatomy	The needle passes through the subcutaneous tissues and penetrates m. rectus capitis posterior major.
Acupuncture	Insert the needle perpendicularly or obliquely 0.5~0.8 cun deep and stimulate until there is a sore and numbing sensation in the local area.

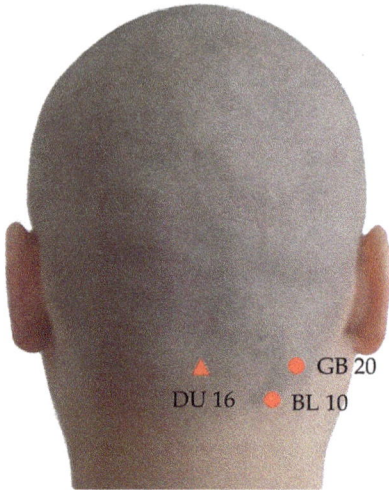

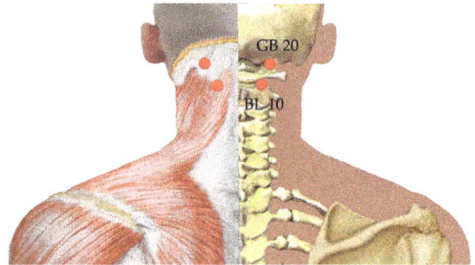

DU-14 — DàZhuī

Position	On the posterior midline of the neck, in the depression inferior to the spinous process of the seventh cervical vertebra.
Acupoint Selection Skills	The point is located in the sitting or prone position when the neck is flexed, in the depression inferior to the spinous process of the seventh cervical vertebra.
Regional Anatomy	The needle passes through the subcutaneous tissues, the supraspinal ligament and interspinal ligament and penetrates the interarcuate ligament.
Acupuncture	Insert the needle perpendicularly 0.8~1.2 cun deep and stimulate until there is a sore and numbing sensation in the local area.

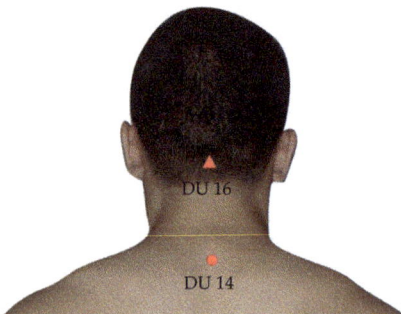

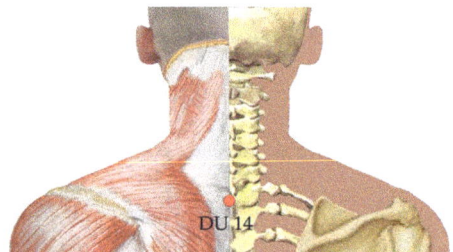

11. EX-HN-3, LI-20, EX-HN-8 — Expels wind and benefits the nose and eyes, activates the collaterals and alleviates pain

Indications	On the face, midway between the medial ends of the two eyebrows.

EX-HN — 3 YìnTáng

Position	On the face, midway between the medial ends of the two eyebrows.
Acupoint Selection Skills	The point is located in the sitting or supine position, at the midpoint of the medial ends of the two eyebrows.
Regional Anatomy	The needle passes through the subcutaneous tissues and penetrates the m. procerus and m. corrugator supercilii and reaches frontal periost.
Acupuncture	Lift and squeeze the skin, insert the needle subcutaneously downwards 0.3~0.5 cun deep and stimulate until there is a sore and distending sensation in the local area.

LI-20 — YíngXiāng

Position	At the middle point of the lateral side of the nostril in the nasolabial groove.
Acupoint Selection Skills	The point is located in the sitting or supine position, at the middle point of the lateral side of the nostril in the nasolabial groove.
Regional Anatomy	The needle passes through the skin, subcutaneous fascia and reaches the m. levatorlabiisuperioris.
Acupuncture	Insert the needle inwards and upwards horizontally 0.5~1.0 cun deep and stimulate until there is a sore and numbing sensation in local area and radiating to the nasal area.

EX-HN — 8 ShàngYíngXiāng

Position	At the junction of the nasal alar cartilage and turbinalia, highest point of the nasolabial groove.
Acupoint Selection Skills	The point is located in the sitting or supine position, at the highest point of the nasolabial groove, 1.5 cun posterior to the LI 20.
Regional Anatomy	The needle passes through the subcutaneous tissues and reaches m. levatorlabii superior isalaequenasi near the facial artery and vein.
Acupuncture	Insert the needle subcutaneously upward 0.5-0.8 cun deep and stimulate until there is a sore and distending sensation in the local area and radiating to the nasal area.

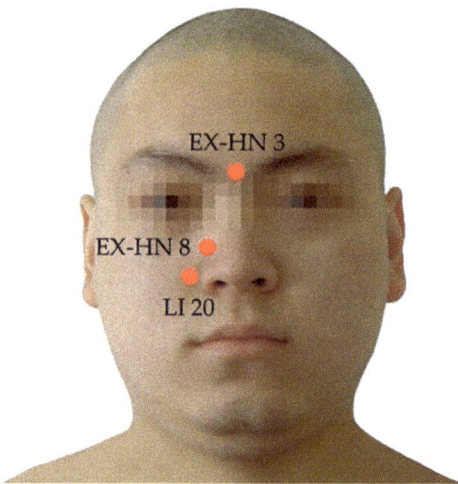

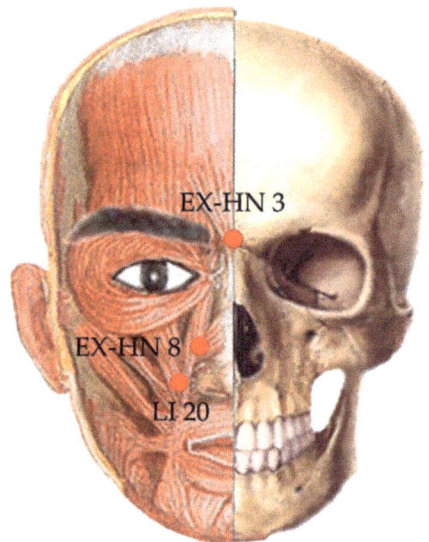

12. EX-HN-5, ST-7, ST-5 — Expels wind and activates collaterals, reduces swelling and alleviates pain

Indications	Headache and dizziness, deviation of the eye and mouth, swelling of the face.

EX-HN — 5 TàiYáng

Position	In the depression about one finger breadth posterior to the midpoint between the lateral end of the eyebrow and the outer canthus.
Acupoint Selection Skills	The point is located in the sitting or supine position, in the depression about one finger breadth posterior to the midpoint between the lateral end of the eyebrow and the outer canthus.
Regional Anatomy	The needle passes through the subcutaneous tissues and penetrates the m. temporalis near the superficial temporal artery and vein.
Acupuncture	① Insert the needle perpendicularly 0.3~0.5 cun deep and stimulate until there is a sore and distending sensation in the local area. ② Insert the needle backwards subcutaneously towards GB 8 1.0~2.0 cun deep and stimulate until there is a sore and distending sensation in the local area radiating to the temporal side.

ST-7 — XiàGuān

Position	In the depression between the zygomatic arch and mandibular notch in front of the ear.
Acupoint Selection Skills	The point is located in the sitting or recumbent position, on the inferior border of the zygomatic arch, anterior to the condyloid process of the mandible.
Regional Anatomy	The needle passes through the posterior aspect of the parotid, penetrates the tendo m. temporalis, and enters infratemporal fossa.
Acupuncture	Insert the needle perpendicularly 1.0~1.5 cun deep and stimulate until there is a sore and numbing sensation in the local area.

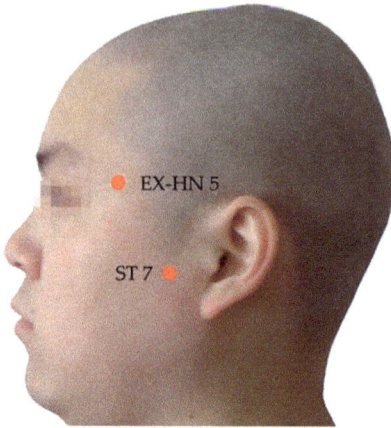

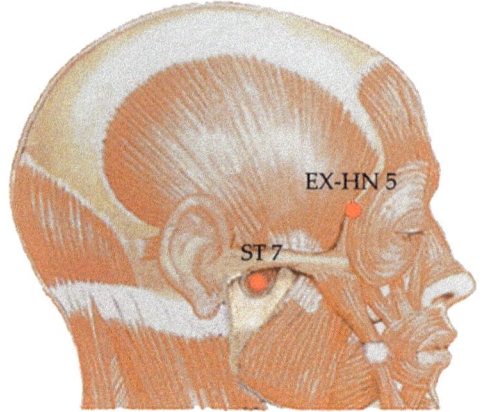

ST-5 — DàYíng

Position	On the lateral side of the face, 1.3 cun anterior and inferior to the corner of the jaw, on the anterior part of the masseter muscle where the pulse of the facial artery can be felt.
Acupoint Selection Skills	The point is located in the sitting or supine position, in the depression in front of the jaw bone where the pulse can be felt.
Regional Anatomy	The needle passes through the subcutaneous tissues, penetrates m. depressor angulioris, and reaches the anterior border of masseter.
Acupuncture	Insert the needle perpendicularly 0.2~0.5 cun deep and stimulate until there is a sore and numbing sensation in the local area radiating to the lateral aspect of the face.

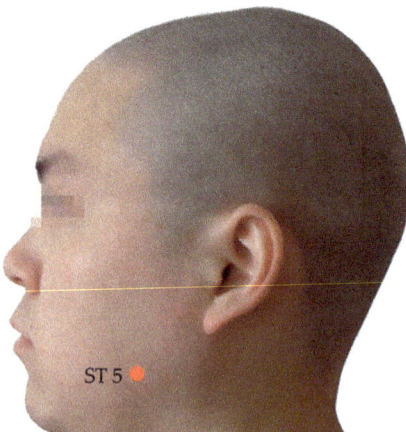

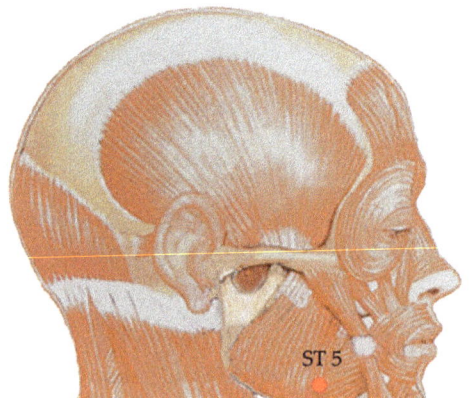

CHAPTER 3

Trunk Combination Points

1. RN-10, RN-12, RN-13 — Invigorates spleen and harmonizes stomach

Indications	Diarrhea, abdominal distention, borbory gums and abdominal pain, indigestion, vomiting, hiccup singultation.

RN-10 — XiàWǎn

Position	On the upper abdomen, on the anterior midline, 2 cun above the umbilicus.
Regional Anatomy	The needle passes through subcutis and penetrates the internal abdominal fascia and subperiotoneal fascia.
Acupuncture	Insert the needle perpendicularly 0.5~1.0 cun deep and stimulate until there is a sore and distending sensation in the local area.

RN-12 — ZhōngWǎn

Position	On the upper abdomen, on the anterior midline, 4 cun superior to the umbilicus.
Regional Anatomy	The needle passes through subcutis and penetrates the internal abdominal fascia and subperiotoneal fascia.
Acupuncture	Insert the needle perpendicularly 0.5~1.0 cun deep and stimulate until there is a sore and distending sensation in the local area radiating to the stomach.

RN-13 — ShàngWǎn

Position	On the upper abdomen, on the anterior midline, 5 cun superior to the umbilicus.
Regional Anatomy	The needle passes through subcutis and penetrates the internal abdominal fascia and subperiotoneal fascia.
Acupuncture	Insert the needle perpendicularly 0.5~1.0 cun deep and stimulate until there is a sore and distending sensation in the local area radiating to the upper abdomen.

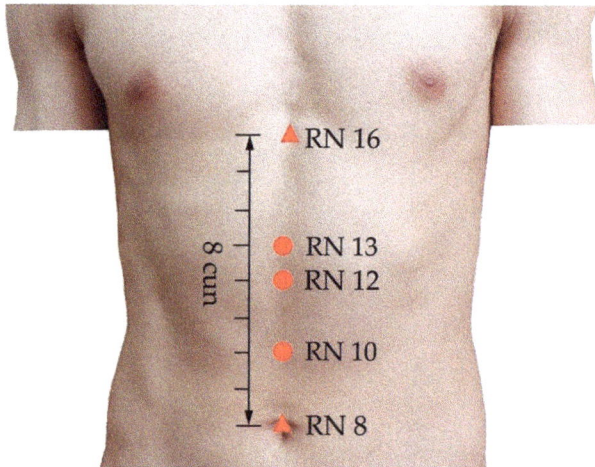

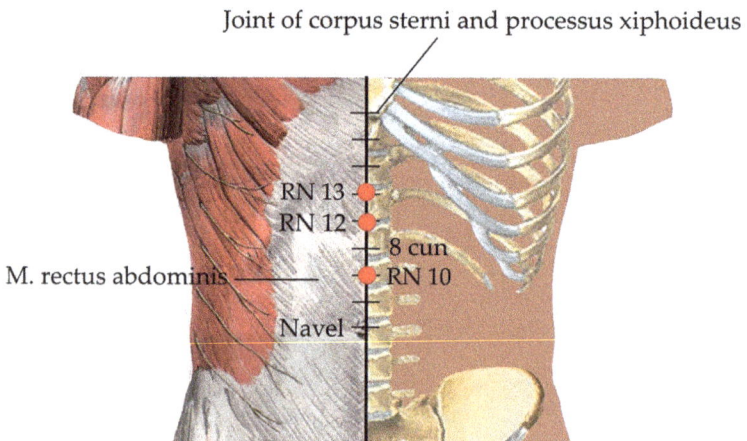

2. RN-4, RN-6 — Tonifies original Qi and benefits essence, tonifies and nourishes kidney, regulates menstruation and leucorrhea, fortifies yang and rescues collapse.

Indications	Abdominal diseases, women's diseases, gastrointestinal diseases, general weakness.

RN-4 — GuānYuán

Position	On the lower abdomen, on the anterior midline, 3 cun inferior to the umbilicus.
Regional Anatomy	The needle passes through the skin and subcutis and penetrates the transverse fascia and median umbilical fold.
Acupuncture	Request for the patient to empty their bladder before the puncturing this point. Insert the needle perpendicularly 0.5~1.0 cun deep and stimulate until there is a sore and distending sensation in the local area radiating to the genitalia. This point can be moxibusted.

RN-6 — QìHǎi

Position	On the lower abdomen, on the anterior midline, 1.5 cun inferior to the umbilicus.
Regional Anatomy	The needle passes through the skin and subcutis, and penetrates the internal abdominal fascia and median umbilical fold.
Acupuncture	Insert the needle perpendicularly 0.8~1.2 cun deep and stimulate until there is a sore and distending sensation in the local area radiating to the genitalia.

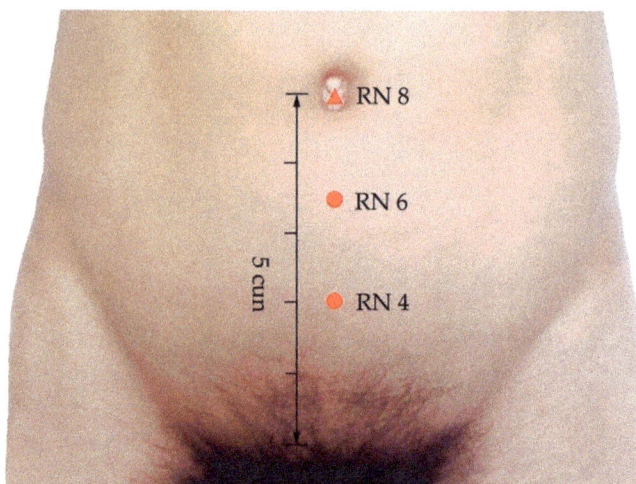

RN 8

RN 6

RN 4

5 cun

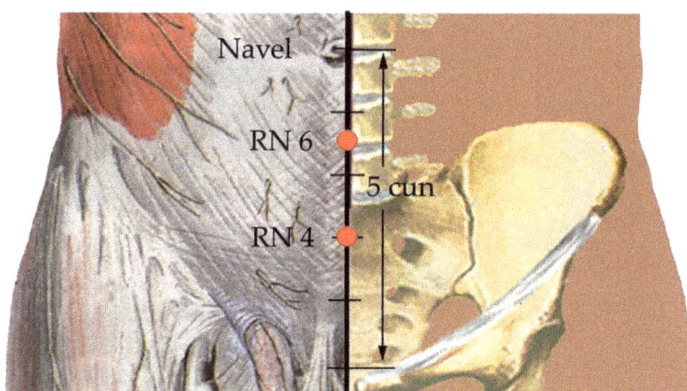

Navel

RN 6

5 cun

RN 4

Acupuncture of Acupoint Combination

3. LV-14, LV-13, GB-25 — Spreads liver and Invigorates spleen, regulates Qi and alleviates pain.

Indications	Distention of the chest and hypochondrium, abdominal distention, vomiting, hiccup singultation, diarrhea, edema, adverse urination.

LV-14 — QīMén

Position	On the chest, directly inferior to the nipple, in the sixth intercostal space, 4 cun lateral to the anterior midline.
Acupoint Selection Skills	The point is located in the supine position, two inter-costal space inferior to ST 17, in the sixth intercostal space, inferior to the mid-clavicle line. For women, the point is located in the clavicles midline, in the sixth intercostal space.
Regional Anatomy	The needle passes through the subcutaneous tissues and penetrates endothoracic fascia.
Acupuncture	Insert the needle obliquely 0.5~0.8 cun deep and stimulate until there is a sore and numbing sensation in the local area radiating to the back.

LV-13 — ZhāngMén

Position	On the lateral aspect of the abdomen, below the free end of the eleventh floating rib.
Acupoint Selection Skills	The point is located in the supine or lateral position, on the mid-axillary line when the elbow is adducted and flexed, at the point under the tip of the elbow.
Regional Anatomy	The needle passes through the subcutaneous tissues and penetrates the subperiotoneal fascia.
Acupuncture	Insert the needle obliquely 0.5~0.8 cun deep and stimulate until there is a sore and numbing sensation in the local area radiating to the external genitalia.

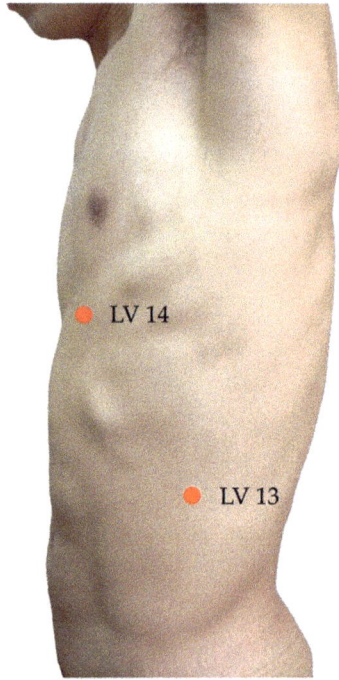

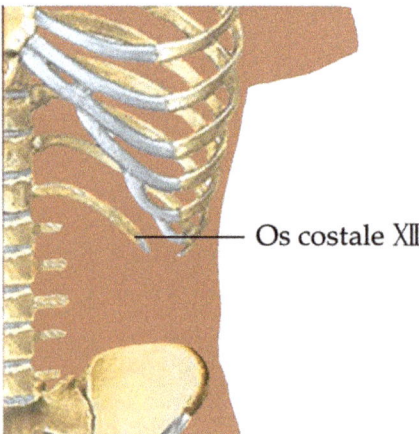

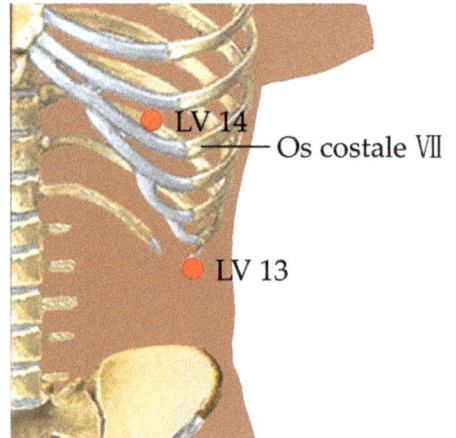

GB-25 — JīngMén

Position	On the lateral aspect of the abdomen, on the lower border of the end of the twelfth floating rib.
Acupoint Selection Skills	The point is located in the lateral position, inferior to the end of the twelfth floating rib.
Regional Anatomy	The needle passes through the subcutaneous tissues and penetrates the subperiotoneal fascia.
Acupuncture	Insert the needle subcutaneously 0.5~1.0 cun deep and stimulate until there is a sore and numbing sensation in the local area radiating to the lower back.

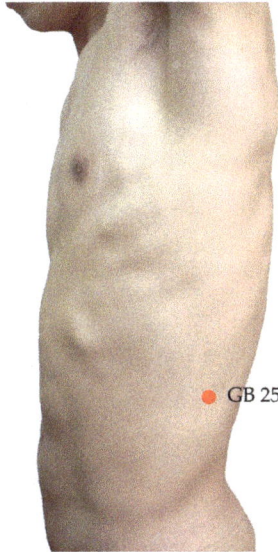

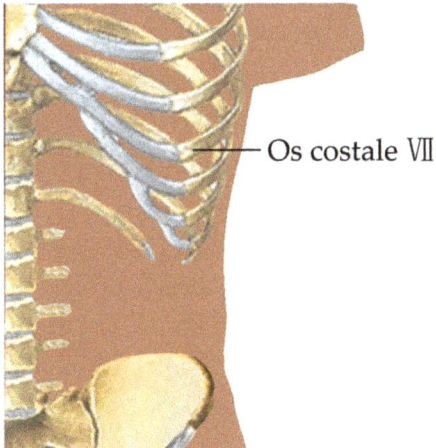

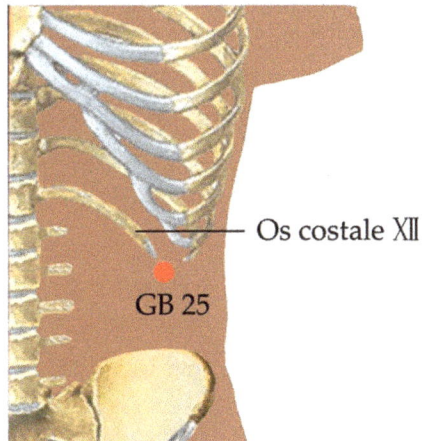

GB 25

Os costale VII

Os costale XII

GB 25

4. KI-25, RN-21 — Unbinds the chest and regulates Qi, alleviates cough and wheezing

Indications	Cough and asthma, pain of the chest, distention of the chest and hypochondrium, sore throat.

KI-25 — ShénCáng

Position	On the chest, in the second intercostal space, 2 cun lateral to the anterior midline.
Acupoint Selection Skills	The point is located in the supine position, in the second intercostal space, 2 cun lateral to the anterior midline.
Regional Anatomy	The needle passes through the skin and subcutaneous tissue, penetrates m. intercostales externi and m. intercostales interni and reaches before the endothoracic fascia.
Acupuncture	Insert the needle obliquely 0.5~0.8 cun deep and stimulate until there is a sore and numbing sensation in the local area radiating to the chest. Avoid deep insertion to prevent injury to the internal organs.

RN-21 — XuánJī

Position	On the chest, on the anterior midline, on the level of the manubrium of the sternum.
Acupoint Selection Skills	The point is located in the sitting or supine position, 1 cun inferior to RN-22.
Regional Anatomy	The needle passes through subcutis and penetrates the periost of presternum.
Acupuncture	Insert the needle subcutaneously 0.3~0.5 cun deep and stimulate until there is a sore and distending sensation in the local area.

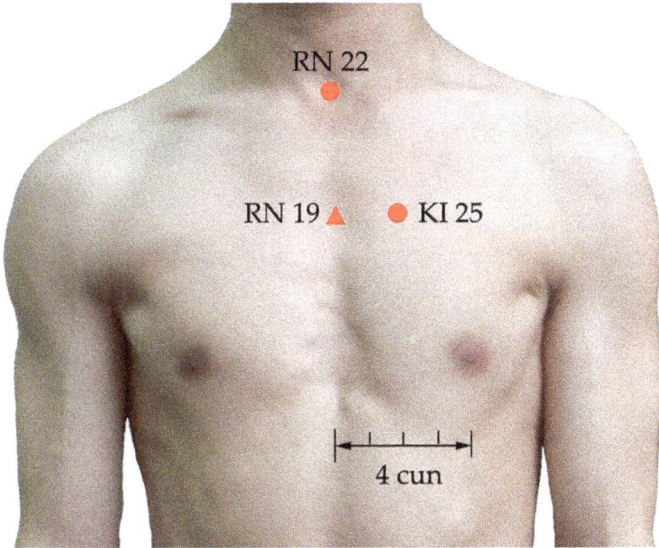

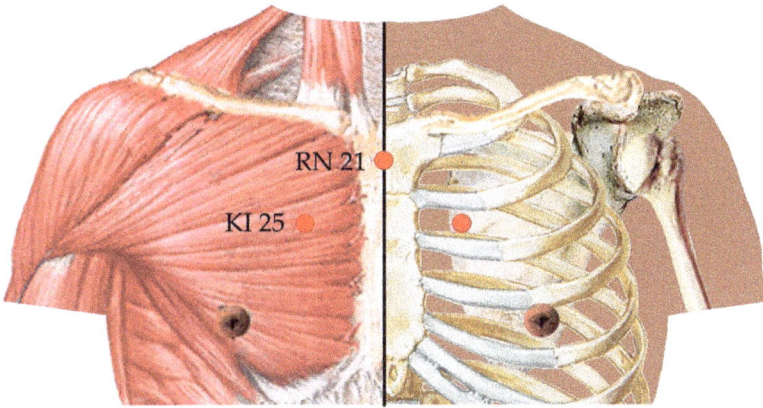

5. RN-12, RN-6, RN-17 — Unbinds the chest and regulates Qi, descends rebellious Qi of the lung and stomach, alleviates cough and wheezing.

Indications	Chest distention, cough, insufficient lactation, hiccup singultation, vomiting, asthma, cardiac pain.

RN-12 — ZhōngWǎn

Position	On the upper abdomen, on the anterior midline, 4 cun superior to the umbilicus.
Regional Anatomy	The needle passes through subcutis and penetrates the internal abdominal fascia and subperiotoneal fascia.
Acupuncture	Insert the needle perpendicularly 0.5~1.0 cun deep and stimulate until there is a sore and distending sensation in the local area radiating to the stomach.

RN-6 — QìHǎi

Position	On the lower abdomen, on the anterior midline, 1.5 cun inferior to the umbilicus.
Regional Anatomy	The needle passes through the skin and subcutis, and penetrates the internal abdominal fascia and median umbilical fold.
Acupuncture	Insert the needle perpendicularly 0.8~1.2 cun deep and stimulate until there is a sore and distending sensation in the local area radiating to the genitalia.

RN-17 — DànZhōng

Position	On the chest, on the anterior midline, at the level of the fourth intercostal space.
Acupoint Selection Skills	The point is located in the supine position, at the junction of the line connecting the two nipples and the midline of the sternum, at the level with the fourth intercostal space.
Regional Anatomy	The needle passes through subcutis and penetrates the periost of sternal body.
Acupuncture	Insert the needle subcutaneously or obliquely 0.3~0.5 cun deep and stimulate until there is a sore and distending sensation in the local area radiating to the chest.

RN 17
RN 16

8 cun

RN 12

RN 8
RN 6

5 cun

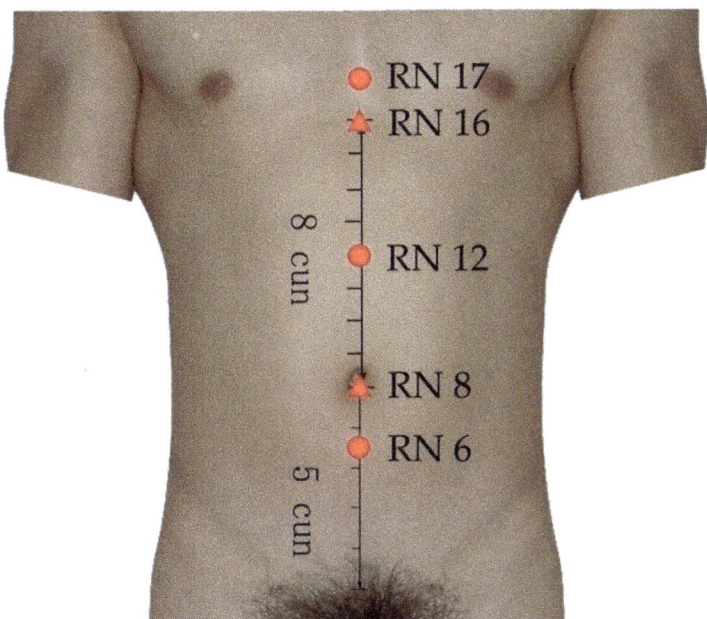

Joint of corpus sterni and processus xiphoideus

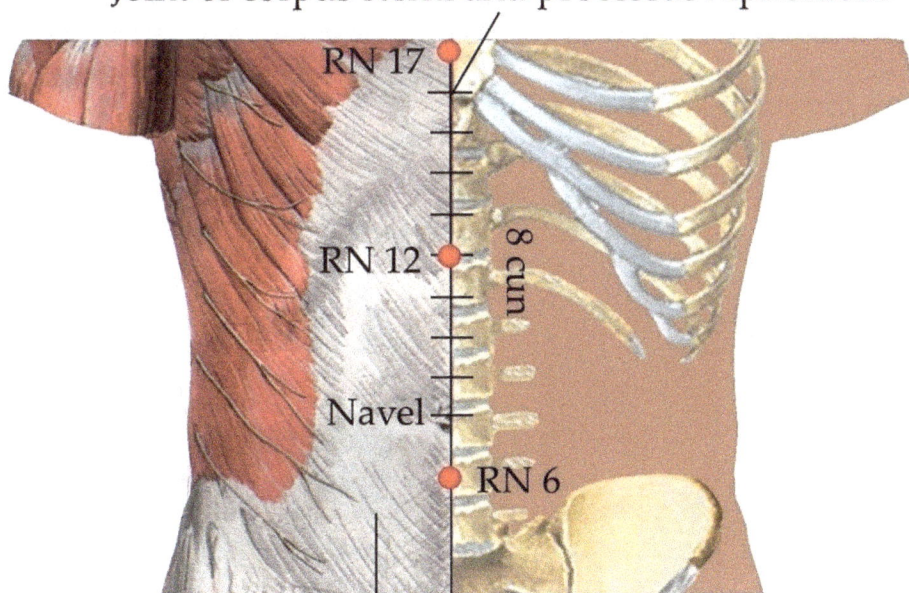

RN 17

8 cun

RN 12

Navel

RN 6

M. rectus abdominis

6. RN-4, ST-25 — Warms middle jiao and harmonizes stomach, regulates Qi and invigorates spleen

(Jiao, has been divided into three parts: upper Jiao, middle Jiao and lower Jiao. Upper Jiao refers mainly to the heart and lung part, middle Jiao refers mainly to the spleen and stomach, lower Jiao refers mainly to liver, bladder and gut.)

Indications	Vomiting, abdominal distention, pain around the umbilicus, constipation, diarrhea, dysentery, indigestion.

RN-4 — GuānYuán

Position	On the lower abdomen, on the anterior midline, 3 cun inferior to the umbilicus.
Regional Anatomy	The needle passes through the skin and subcutis and penetrates the transverse fascia and median umbilical fold.
Acupuncture	Request the patient empties their bladder before the puncturing this point. Insert the needle perpendicularly 0.5~1.0 cun deep and stimulate until there is a sore and distending sensation in the local area radiating to the genitalia. This point can be moxibusted.

ST-25 — TiānShū

Position	On the abdomen, 2 cun lateral to the umbilicus.
Regional Anatomy	The needle passes through the subcutaneous tissues and penetrates the posterior layer of sheath of m. rectus abdominis and m. rectus abdominis.
Acupuncture	Insert the needle perpendicularly 1.0~1.5 cun deep and stimulate until there is a sore and numbing sensation in the local area radiating to the side of the abdomen.

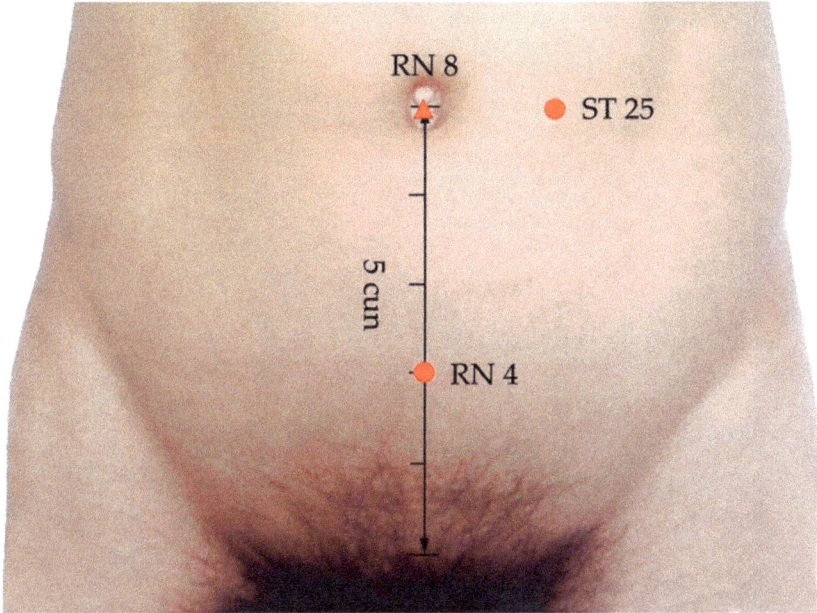

RN 8

ST 25

5 cun

RN 4

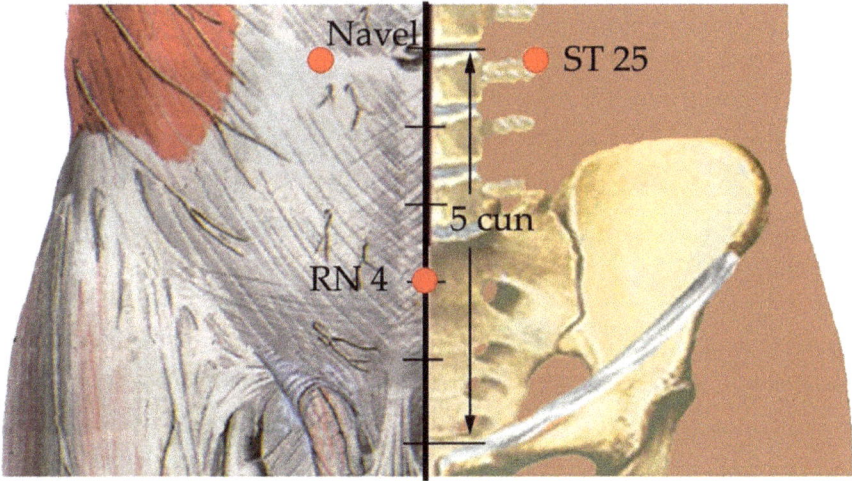

Navel

ST 25

5 cun

RN 4

Symphysis pubica

7. RN-17, LV-14 — Spreads liver and Invigorates spleen, regulates Qi and descends rebellious Qi

Indications	Pain and distention in the hypochondrium, belching, hiccup singultation.

RN-17 — DànZhōng

Position	On the chest, on the anterior midline, at the level of the fourth intercostals space.
Acupoint Selection Skills	The point is located in the supine position, at the junction of the line connecting the two nipples and the midline of the sternum, at the level with the fourth intercostal space.
Regional Anatomy	The needle passes through subcutis and penetrates the periost of the sternal body.
Acupuncture	Insert the needle subcutaneously or obliquely 0.3~0.5 cun deep and stimulate until there is a sore and distending sensation in the local area radiating to the chest.

LV-14 — QīMén

Position	On the chest, directly inferior to the nipple, in the sixth intercostal space, 4 cun lateral to the anterior midline.
Acupoint Selection Skills	The point is located in the supine position, two intercostal space inferior to ST 17, in the sixth intercostal space, inferior to the mid-clavicle line. For women, the point is located in the clavicles midline, in the sixth intercostal space.
Regional Anatomy	The needle passes through the subcutaneous tissues and penetrates endothoracic fascia.
Acupuncture	Insert the needle obliquely 0.5~0.8 cun deep and stimulate until there is a sore and numbing sensation in the local area radiating to the back.

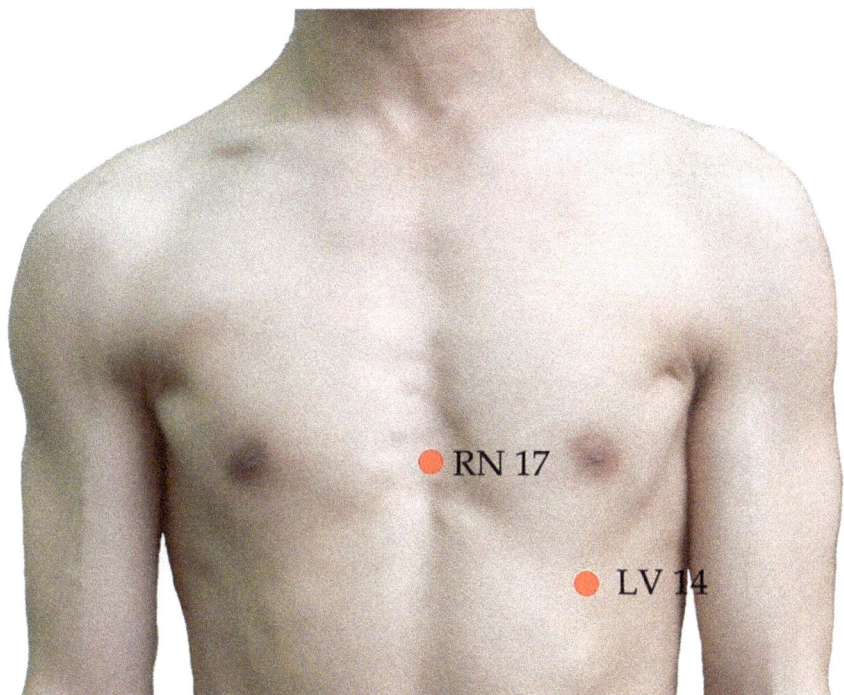

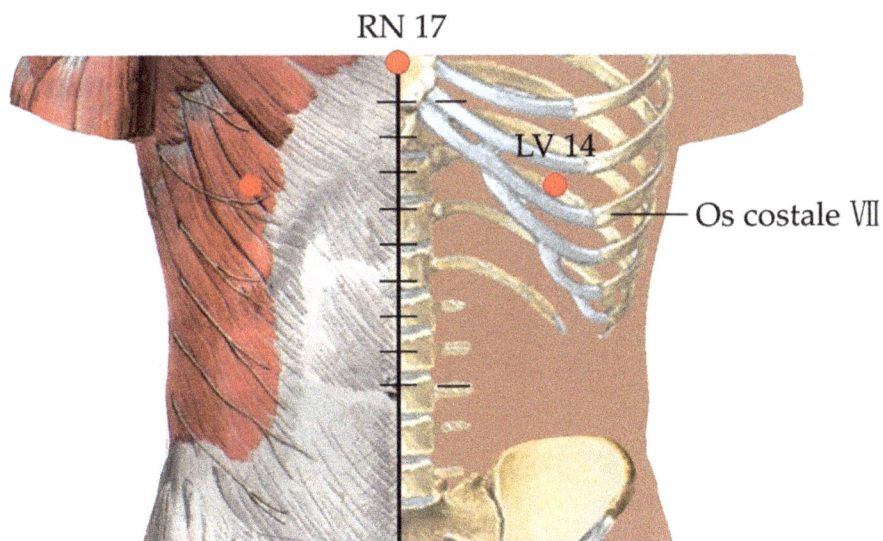

8. RN-4, RN-3, ST-29 — Transforms dampness and clears heat, tonifies kidney and regulates menstruation

Indications	Pain in the lower abdomen, inhibited urination, hernia, perineal pain, pruritus perineum, irregular menstruation, spermatorrhea.

RN-4 — GuānYuán

Position	On the lower abdomen, on the anterior midline, 3 cun inferior to the umbilicus.
Regional Anatomy	The needle passes through the skin and subcutis and penetrates the transverse fascia and median umbilical fold.
Acupuncture	Request the patient empties their bladder before puncturing this point. Insert the needle perpendicularly 0.5~1.0 cun deep and stimulate until there is a sore and distending sensation in the local area radiating to the genitalia.

RN-3 – ZhōngJí

Position	On the lower abdomen, on the anterior midline, 4 cun inferior to the umbilicus.
Regional Anatomy	The needle passes through the skin and subcutis, and penetrates the subperiotoneal fascia and median umbilical fold.
Acupuncture	Request the patient empties their bladder before the puncturing this point. Insert the needle perpendicularly 0.5~1.0 cun deep and stimulate until there is a sore and distending sensation in the local area radiating to the genitalia.

ST-29 – GuīLái

Position	On the lower abdomen, 4 cun inferior to the umbilicus, 2 cun lateral from the anterior midline.
Acupoint Selection Skills	The point is located in the supine position, on the lower abdomen, 2 cun lateral from the ST – 29.
Regional Anatomy	The needle passes through the subcutaneous tissues and penetrates the posterior layer of sheath of m. rectus abdominis, m. rectus abdominis and peritoneum.
Acupuncture	Insert the needle perpendicularly 1.0~1.5 cun deep and stimulate until there is a sore heavy sensation in the lower abdomen.

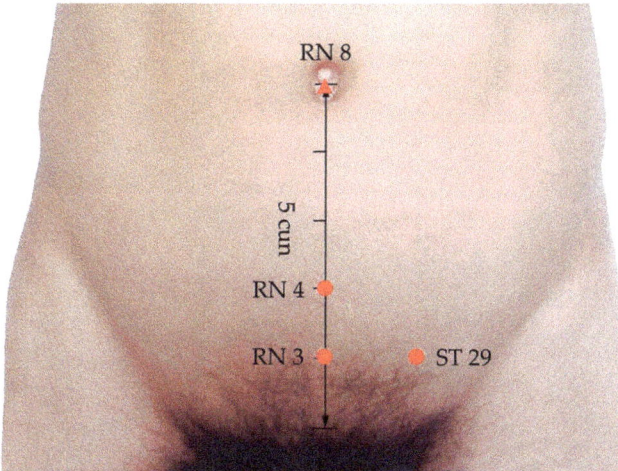

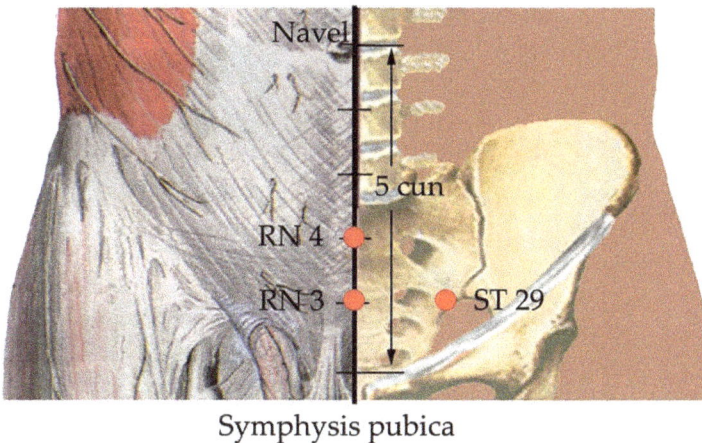

Symphysis pubica

9. DU-14, BL-12, BL-13 — Expels wind and strengthens exterior, disperses and descends lung Qi

Indications	Headache and fever, pain of the shoulder and back, cough and asthma.

DU-14 — DàZhuī

Position	On the posterior midline of the neck, in the depression inferior to the spinous process of the seventh cervical vertebra.
Acupoint Selection Skills	The point is located in the sitting or prone position when the neck is flexed, in the depression inferior to the spinous process of the seventh cervical vertebra.
Regional Anatomy	The needle passes through the subcutaneous tissues, the supraspinal ligament and interspinal ligament and penetrates the interarcuate ligament.
Acupuncture	Insert the needle perpendicularly 0.8~1.2 cun deep and stimulate until there is a sore and numbing sensation in the local area spreading to the shoulder and arm. Avoid deep insertion to prevent injury to the spinal cord.

BL-12 — FēngMén

Position	On the upper back, 1.5 cun lateral to the lower border of the spinous process of the second thoracic vertebra.
Regional Anatomy	The needle passes through the subcutaneous tissues and penetrates m. sacrospinalis.
Acupuncture	Insert the needle obliquely towards the spine 0.5~0.8 cun deep and stimulate until there is a sore and numbing sensation in the local area radiating to the intercostal space.

BL-13 — FèiShū

Position	On the upper back, 1.5 cun lateral to the lower border of the spinous process of the third thoracic vertebra.
Regional Anatomy	The needle passes through the subcutaneous tissues and penetrates m. sacrospinalis.
Acupuncture	Insert the needle obliquely towards the spine 0.5~0.8 cun deep and stimulate until there is a sore and numbing sensation in the local area radiating to the intercostal space. Avoid deep insertion to prevent pneumothorax.

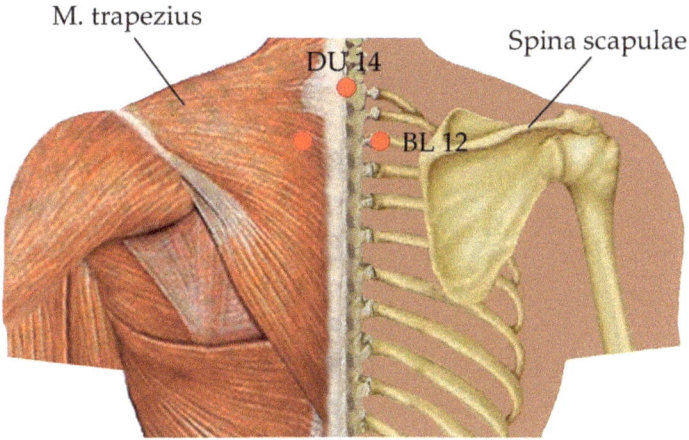

M. trapezius

DU 14

Spina scapulae

BL 12

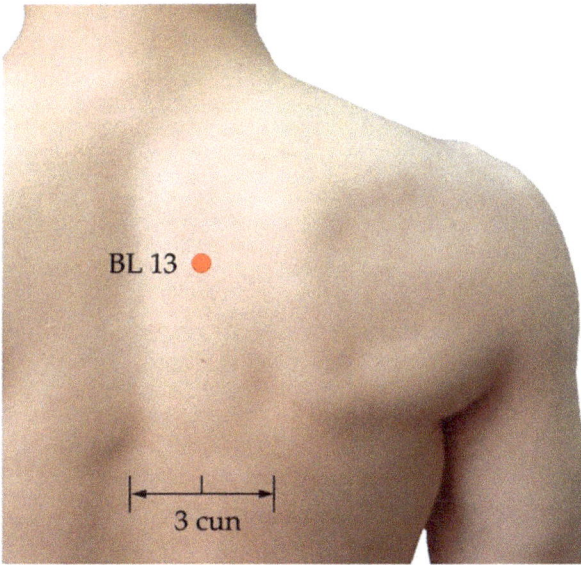

BL 13

3 cun

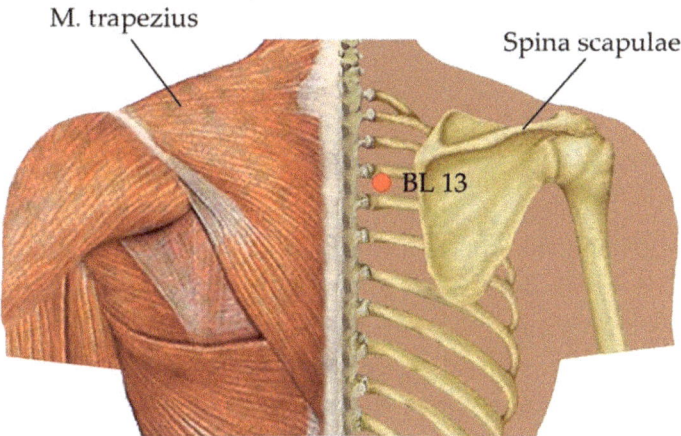

M. trapezius

Spina scapulae

BL 13

10. DU-10, DU-11, BL-15 — Regulates Qi and blood, activates the channel, tonifies heart and calms spirit.

Indications	Asthma, neck stiffness and back pain, easily frightened, cardiac pain and palpitations, insomnia and amnesia, night sweat, nocturnal emission.

DU-10 — LíngTái

Position	On the posterior midline of the back, in the depression inferior to the spinous process of the sixth thoracic vertebra.
Regional Anatomy	The needle passes through the subcutaneous tissues, the supraspinal ligament and interspinal ligament and penetrates the interarcuate ligament.
Acupuncture	Insert the needle perpendicularly or obliquely 0.5~1.0 cun deep and stimulate until there is a sore and numbing sensation in the local area spreading to the back and chest. Avoid deep insertion to prevent injury to the spinal cord.

DU-11 — ShénDào

Position	On the posterior midline of the back, in the depression inferior to the spinous process of the fifth thoracic vertebra.
Regional Anatomy	The needle passes through the subcutaneous tissues, the supraspinal ligament and interspinal ligament, and penetrates the interarcuate ligament.
Acupuncture	Insert the needle obliquely 0.5~1.0 cun deep with the twirling or rotating needling technique and stimulate until there is a sore and numbing sensation in the local area spreading to the back and chest. Avoid deep insertion to prevent injury to the spinal cord.

BL-15 — XīnShū

Position	On the upper back, 1.5 cun lateral to the lower border of the spinous process of the fifth thoracic vertebra.
Regional Anatomy	The needle passes through the subcutaneous tissues and penetrates m. sacrospinalis.
Acupuncture	Insert the needle obliquely towards the spine 0.5~0.8 cun deep and stimulate until there is a sore and numbing sensation in the local area radiating to the intercostal space.

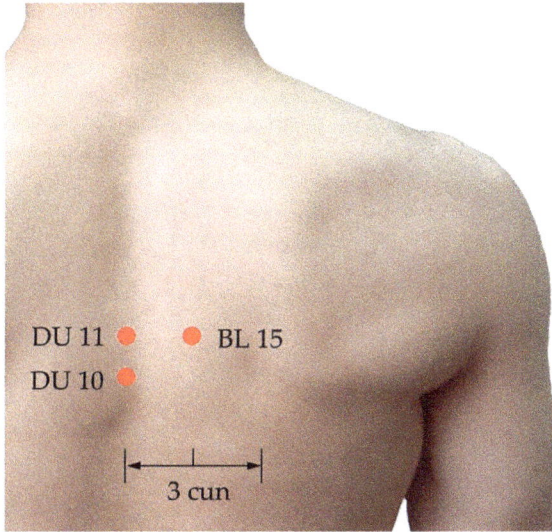

DU 11 BL 15
DU 10

3 cun

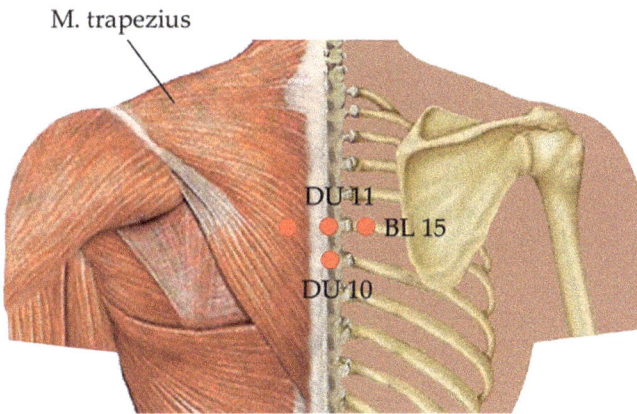

M. trapezius

DU 11
BL 15
DU 10

11. BL-20, BL-21, DU-9 — Invigorates spleen and harmonizes stomach, resolves dampness and promotes digestion

Indications	Abdominal distention, diarrhea, dysentery, stomach-ache, vomiting, lumbago, undigested food, pain in the chest and hypochondriac region, jaundice.

BL-20 — PíShū

Position	On the back, 1.5 cun lateral to the lower border of the spinous process of the eleventh thoracic vertebra.
Regional Anatomy	The needle passes through the subcutaneous tissues and penetrates m. serratus posterior inferior and m. sacrospinalis.
Acupuncture	Insert the needle obliquely towards the spine 0.5~0.8 cun deep and stimulate until there is a sore and numbing sensation in the local area radiating to the intercostal space.

BL-21 — WèiShū

Position	On the back, 1.5 cun lateral to the lower border of the spinous process of the twelfth thoracic vertebra.
Regional Anatomy	The needle passes through the subcutaneous tissues and penetrates m. serratus posterior inferior and m. sacrospinalis.
Acupuncture	Insert the needle perpendicularly 0.5~0.8 cun deep and stimulate until there is a sore and numbing sensation in the local area radiating to the abdomen.

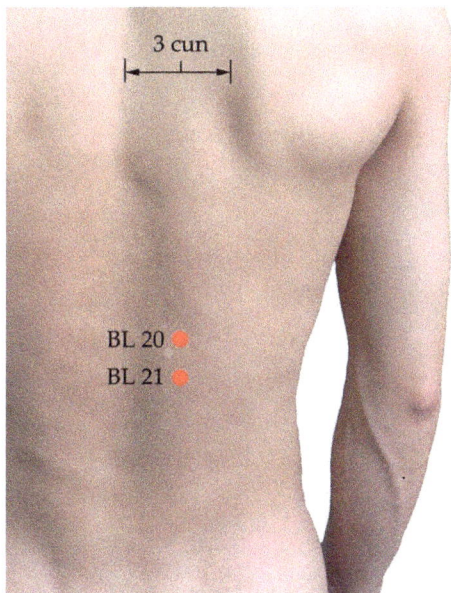

3 cun

BL 20

BL 21

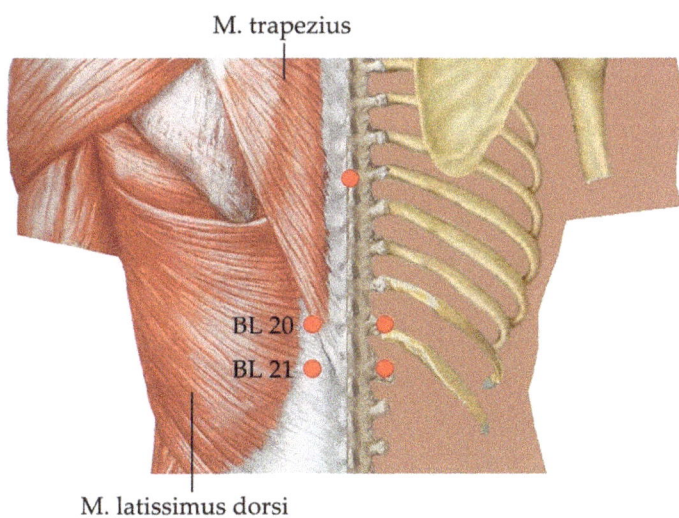

M. trapezius

BL 20

BL 21

M. latissimus dorsi

DU-9 — ZhìYáng

Position	On the posterior midline of the back, in the depression inferior to the spinous process of the seventh thoracic vertebra.
Acupoint Selection Skills	The point is located in the prone position with arm adducted, at the level with the inferior border of the scapula.
Regional Anatomy	The needle passes through the subcutaneous tissues, the supraspinal ligament and interspinal ligament and penetrates the interarcuate ligament.
Acupuncture	Insert the needle perpendicularly or obliquely 0.5~1.0 cun deep and stimulate until there is a sore and numbing sensation in the local area spreading to the back and chest. Avoid deep insertion to prevent injury to the spinal cord.

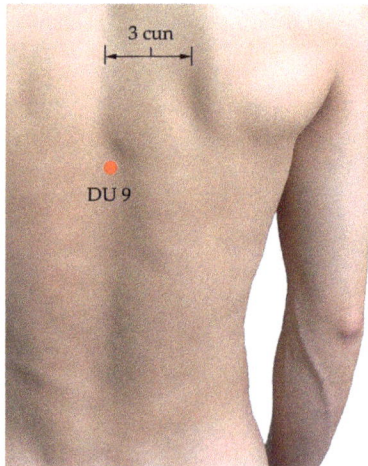

3 cun

DU 9

M. trapezius

DU 9

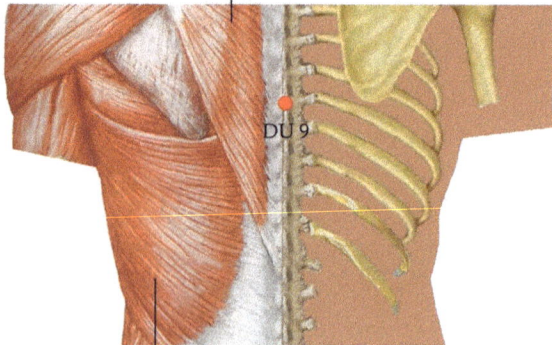

M. latissimus dorsi

12. BL-17, BL-19 — Regulates Qi and descends rebellious Qi, activates blood circulation and collaterals, spreads liver and regulates gall bladder

BL-17 — GéShū

Position	On the back, 1.5 cun lateral to the lower border of the spinous process of the seventh thoracic vertebra.
Acupoint Selection Skills	The point is located in the prone position, at the level with the inferior border of the spinous process of the seventh thoracic vertebra, 1.5 cun lateral to DU – 9, at the level with the inferior edge of the scapula.
Regional Anatomy	The needle passes through the subcutaneous tissues and penetrates m. latissimus dorsi and m. sacrospinalis.
Acupuncture	Insert the needle obliquely towards the spine 0.5~0.8 cun deep and stimulate until there is a sore and numbing sensation in the local area radiating to the intercostal space. Avoid deep insertion to prevent pneumothorax.

BL-19 — DănShū

Position	On the back, 1.5 cun lateral to the lower border of the spinous process of the tenth thoracic vertebra.
Regional Anatomy	The needle passes through the subcutaneous tissues and penetrates m. serratus posterior inferior and m. sacrospinalis.
Acupuncture	Insert the needle obliquely towards the spine 0.5~0.8 cun deep and stimulate until there is a sore and numbing sensation in the local area radiating to the intercostal space. Avoid deep insertion to prevent pneumothorax.

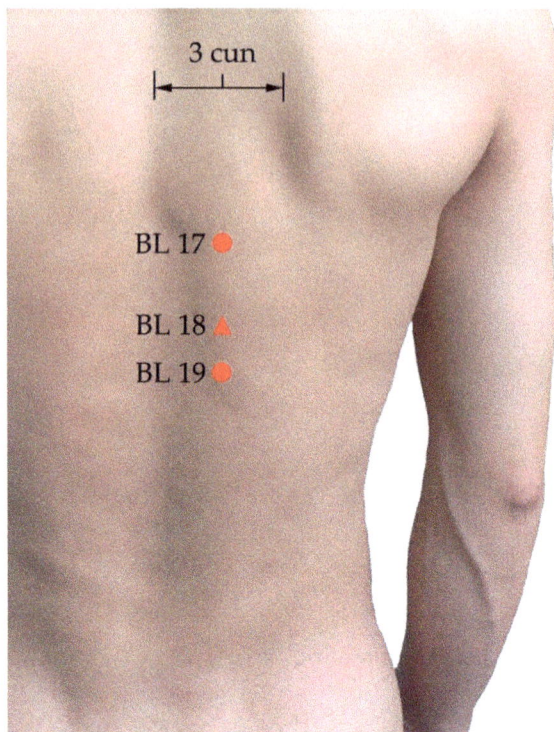

3 cun

BL 17

BL 18

BL 19

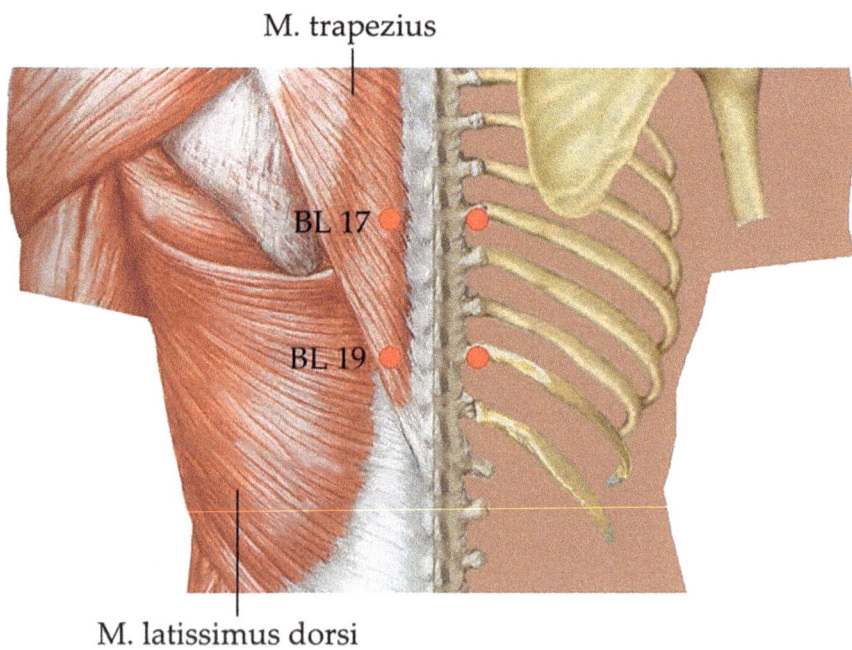

M. trapezius

BL 17

BL 19

M. latissimus dorsi

13. DU-8, BL-18 — Spreads liver and fortifies yang, regulates Qi and calms spirit

(Yin and Yang of human body: those visible/ material parts, skin, muscle, vein, neuro – the whole body is considered as yin, while the power/ function of the body refers to yang, like we could lift thing, digest, excrete mucus, in a word, metabolism. So the "forties yang" of this part refers to strengthen the power of human body and the functions of organs.)

Indications	Abdominal distention, chest congestion, jaundice, indigestion, convulsion, spasms and stiffness of the back, epilepsy.

DU-8 — JīnSuō

Position	On the posterior midline of the back, in the depression inferior to the spinous process of the ninth thoracic vertebra.
Regional Anatomy	The needle passes through the subcutaneous tissues, the supraspinal ligament and interspinal ligament and penetrates the interarcuate ligament.
Acupuncture	Insert the needle obliquely 0.5~1.0 cun deep and stimulate with the twirling or rotating needling technique until there is a sore and numbing sensation in the local area.

BL-18 — GānShū

Position	On the back, 1.5 cun lateral to the lower border of the spinous process of the ninth thoracic vertebra.
Regional Anatomy	The needle passes through the subcutaneous tissues and penetrates m. latissimus dorsi and m. sacrospinalis.
Acupuncture	Insert the needle obliquely towards the spine 0.5~0.8 cun deep and stimulate until there is a sore and numbing sensation in the local area radiating to the intercostal space. Avoid deep insertion to prevent pneumothorax.

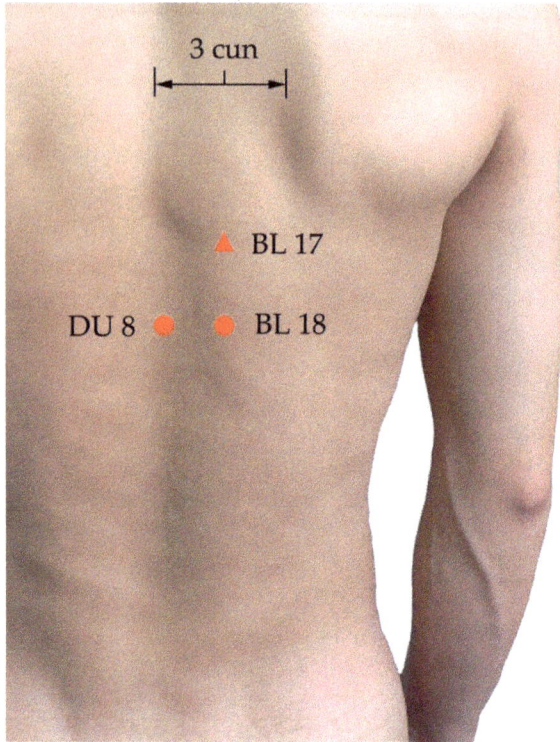

3 cun

▲ BL 17

DU 8 ● ● BL 18

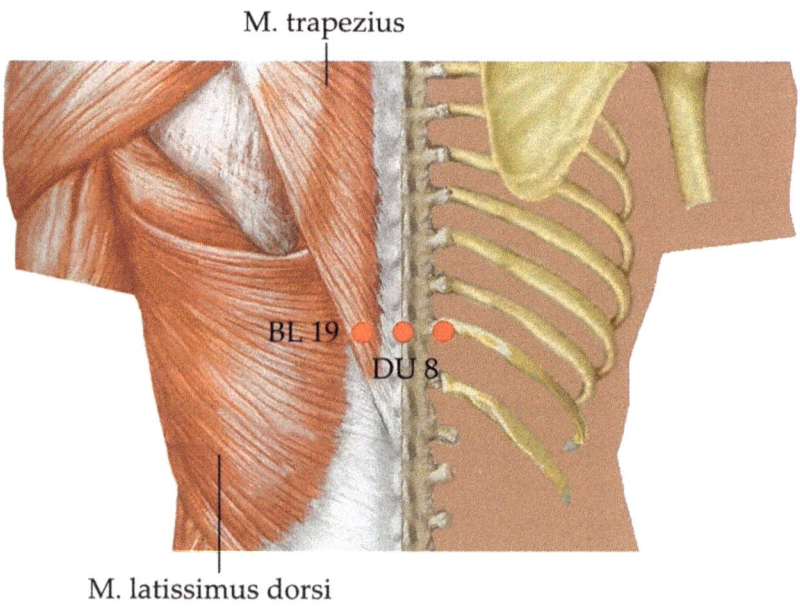

M. trapezius

BL 19 ● ● ●
DU 8

M. latissimus dorsi

14. BL-18, DU-4 — Fortifies yang and benefits essence, tonifies original Qi and tonifies kidney

Indications	Spermatorrhea, impotence, nuresis and dysuria, infertility, stiffness and pain of the lumbar and lower limbs, night blindness, blurred vision.

BL-18 — GānShū

Position	On the back, 1.5 cun lateral to the lower border of the spinous process of the ninth thoracic vertebra.
Regional Anatomy	The needle passes through the subcutaneous tissues and penetrates m. latissimus dorsi and m. sacrospinalis.
Acupuncture	Insert the needle obliquely towards the spine 0.5~0.8 cun deep and stimulate until there is a sore and numbing sensation in the local area radiating to the intercostal space. Avoid deep insertion to prevent pneumothorax.

DU-4 — MìngMén

Position	On the lumbar region, on the posterior midline, in the depression inferior to the spinous process of the second lumbar vertebra.
Acupoint Selection Skills	The point is located in the prone position, two spinous processes above DU 3, on the opposite side of the umbilicus.
Regional Anatomy	The needle passes through the subcutaneous tissues, the supraspinal ligament and interspinal ligament and penetrates the interarcuate ligament.
Acupuncture	Insert the needle perpendicularly or obliquely 0.5~1.0 cun deep and stimulate until there is a sore and numbing sensation in the local area with an electric sensation radiating to the hip and lower limbs. Avoid deep insertion to prevent injury to the spinal cord.

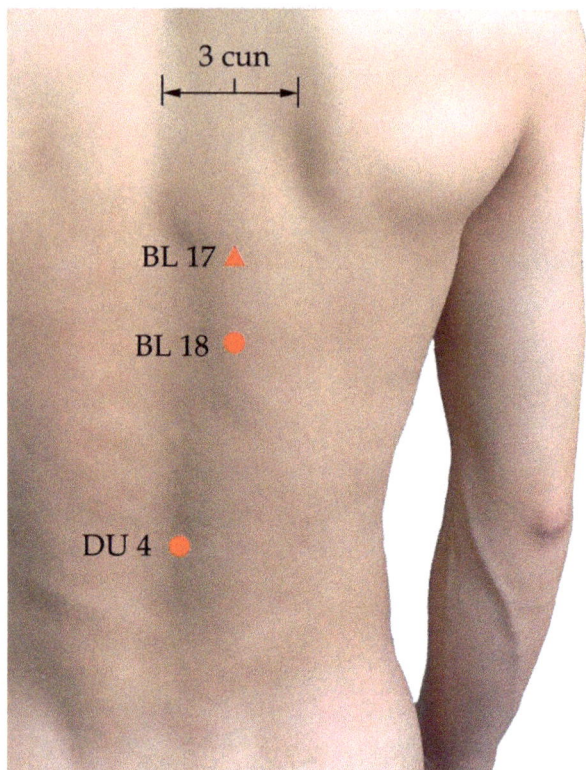

3 cun

BL 17

BL 18

DU 4

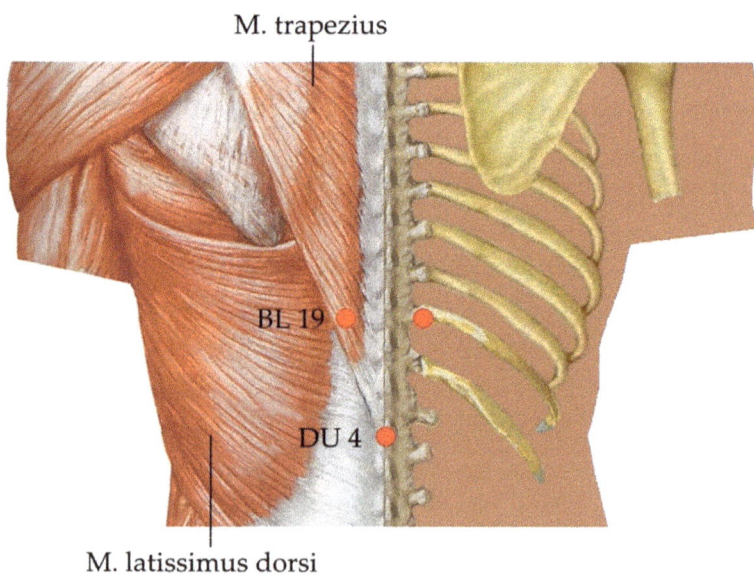

M. trapezius

BL 19

DU 4

M. latissimus dorsi

15. BL-23, DU-4, DU-3 — Benefits original Qi, strenthens kidney Qi and lumbar region

Indications	Pain of the lumbosacral region, weakness and numbness of the limbs, irregular menstruation, spermatorrhea, impotence.

BL-23 — ShènShū

Position	On the lower back, 1.5 cun lateral to the lower border of the spinous process of the second lumbar vertebra.
Acupoint Selection Skills	The point is located in the prone position, at the level with the inferior border of the spinous process of the second lumbar vertebra, 1.5 cun lateral to DU-4 on the opposite side of RN-8.
Regional Anatomy	The needle passes through the subcutaneous tissues and penetrates m. quadratus lumborum and m. psoas major.
Acupuncture	Insert the needle perpendicularly 0.5~1.0 cun deep and stimulate until there is a sore and numbing sensation in the local area radiating to the hip and down the leg.

DU-4 — MìngMén

Position	On the lumbar region, on the posterior midline, in the depression inferior to the spinous process of the second lumbar vertebra.
Acupoint Selection Skills	The point is located in the prone position, two spinous processes above DU-3, on the opposite side of the umbilicus.
Regional Anatomy	The needle passes through the subcutaneous tissues, the supraspinal ligament and interspinal ligament and penetrates the interarcuate ligament.
Acupuncture	Insert the needle perpendicularly or obliquely 0.5~1.0 cun deep and stimulate until there is a sore and numbing sensation in the local area with an electric sensation radiating to the hip and lower limbs. Avoid deep insertion to prevent injury to the spinal cord.

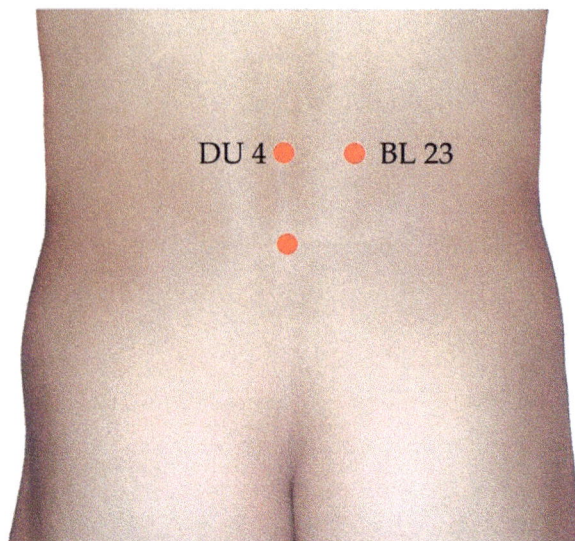

M. latissimus dorsi

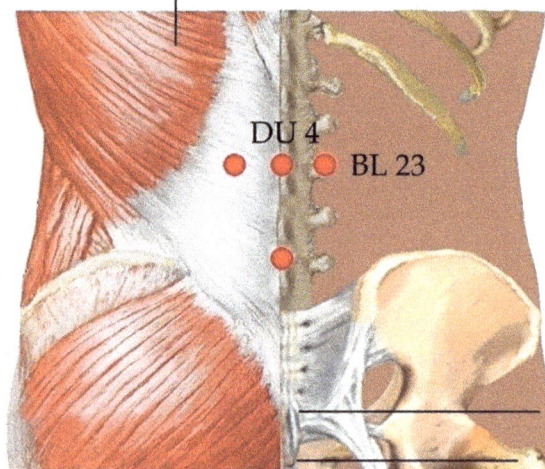

DU-3 — YāoYángGuān

Position	On the lumbar region, on the posterior midline, in the depression inferior to the spinous process of the fourth lumbar vertebra.
Acupoint Selection Skills	The point is located in the prone position, in the depression inferior to the spinous process of the fourth lumbar vertebra at the level with the crista iliaca.

Regional Anatomy	The needle passes through the subcutaneous tissues and supraspinal ligament and penetrates the interarcuate ligament.
Acupuncture	Insert the needle perpendicularly or obliquely 0.5~1.0 cun deep and stimulate until there is a sore and numbing sensation in the local area radiating to the lower limbs.

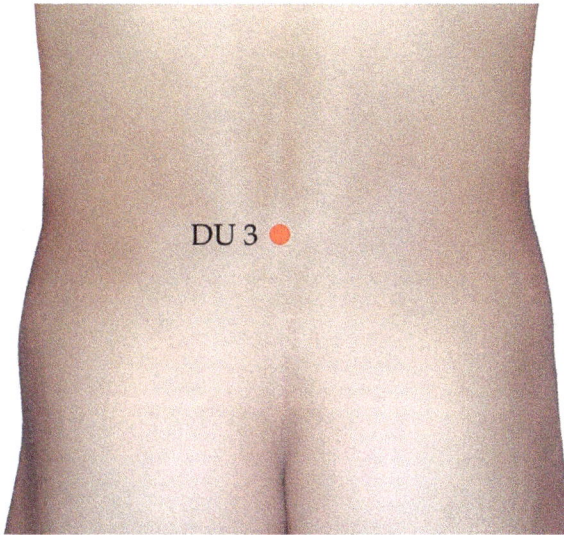

M. latissimus dorsi

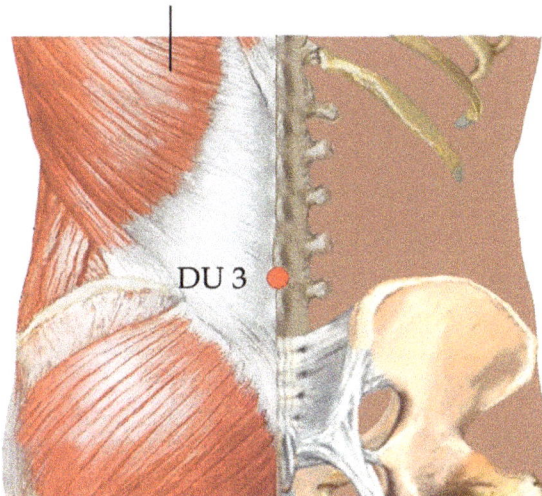

16. BL-28, BL-23 — Strenthens kidney and lumbar region, fortifies yang and benefits urination

Indications	Spermatorrhea, impotence, enuresis, irregular menstruation, morbid leucorrhea, infertility, dysuria, edema.

BL-28 — PángGuāngShū

Position	On the sacrum, 1.5 cun lateral to the middle of the sacral crest, at the level with the second posterior sacral foramen.
Acupoint Selection Skills	The point is located in the prone position, 1.5 cun lateral to the middle of the sacral crest, at the level with the second posterior sacral foramen.
Regional Anatomy	The needle passes through the subcutaneous tissues and penetrates m. latissimus dorsi andm. sacrospinalis.
Acupuncture	Insert the needle perpendicularly 0.8~1.0 cun deep and stimulate until there is a sore and numbing sensation in the local area radiating to the hip and down the leg.

BL-23 — ShènShū

Position	On the lower back, 1.5 cun lateral to the lower border of the spinous process of the second lumbar vertebra.
Acupoint Selection Skills	The point is located in the prone position, at the level with the inferior border of the spinous process of the second lumbar vertebra, 1.5 cun lateral to DU-4 on the opposite side of RN-8.
Regional Anatomy	The needle passes through the subcutaneous tissues and penetrates m. quadratus lumborum and m. psoas major.
Acupuncture	Insert the needle perpendicularly 0.5~1.0 cun deep and stimulate until there is a sore and numbing sensation in the local area radiating to the hip and down the leg.

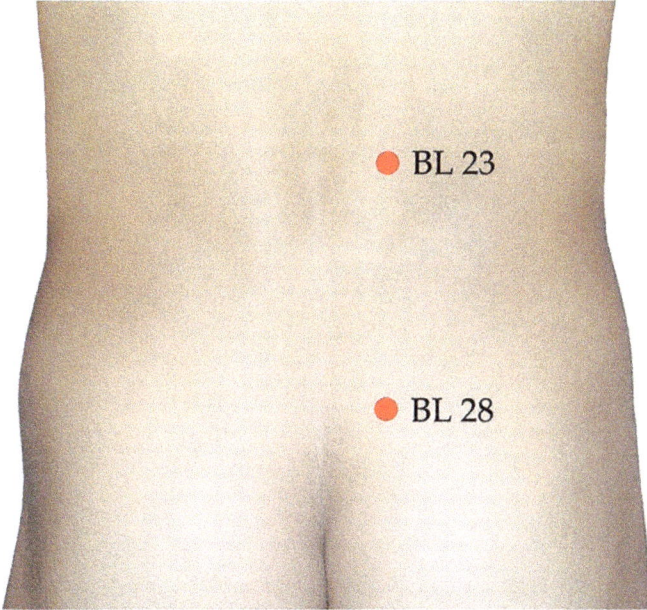

M. latissimus dorsi

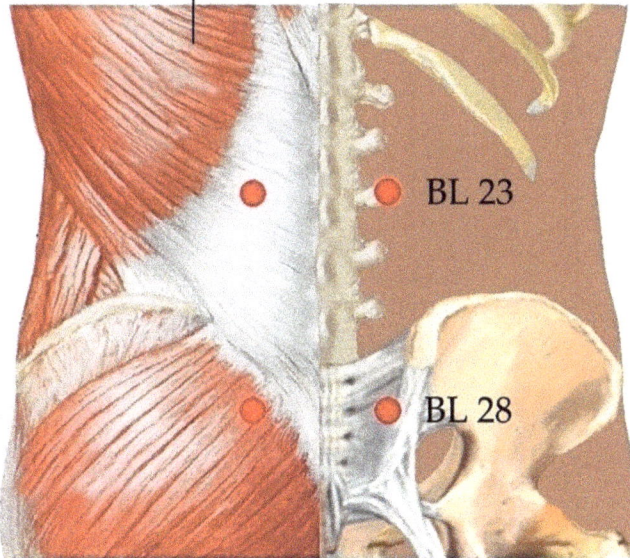

BL 23

BL 28

17. BL-25, BL-54 — Tonifies the lumbar region and lower limbs, activates the channel and activates collaterals, regulates lower jiao

Indications	Pain of the lumbosacral region, weakness and numbness of the limbs, hemorrhoids, constipation, dysuria.

BL-25 — DàChángShū

Position	On the lower back, 1.5 cun lateral to the lower border of the spinous process of the fourth lumbar vertebra.
Regional Anatomy	The needle passes through the subcutaneous tissues and penetrates m. quadratus lumborum and m. psoas major.
Acupuncture	Insert the needle perpendicularly 0.5~0.8 cun deep and stimulate until there is a sore and numbing sensation in the local area radiating to the hip and down the leg.

BL-54 — ZhìBiān

Position	On the lower back, 3 cun lateral to the middle sacral creast, at the level with the fourth posterior sacral foramen.
Acupoint Selection Skills	The point is located in the prone position, 3 cun lateral to the fourth posterior sacral foramen, at the level with the sacral crevice.
Regional Anatomy	The needle passes through the subcutaneous tissues and penetrates m. gluteus maximus.
Acupuncture	Insert the needle perpendicularly obliquely 1.5~3.0 cun deep and stimulate until there is a sore and numbing sensation in the local area radiating to the lower abdomen and hips.

DU 3 ▲ ● BL 25

● BL 54

● BL 25

● BL 54

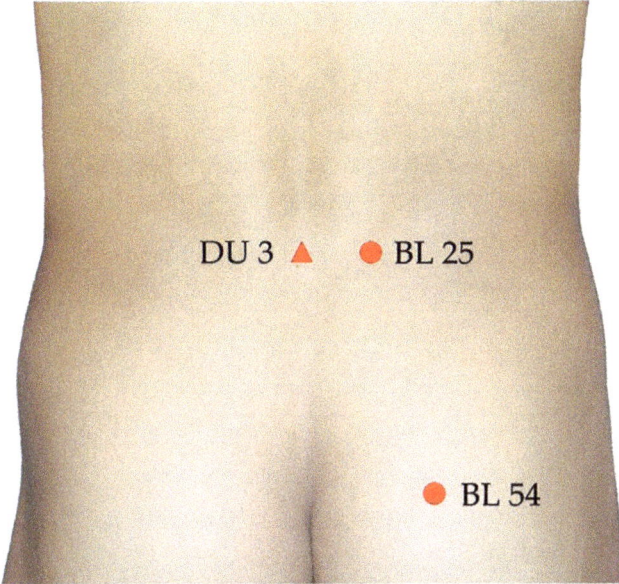

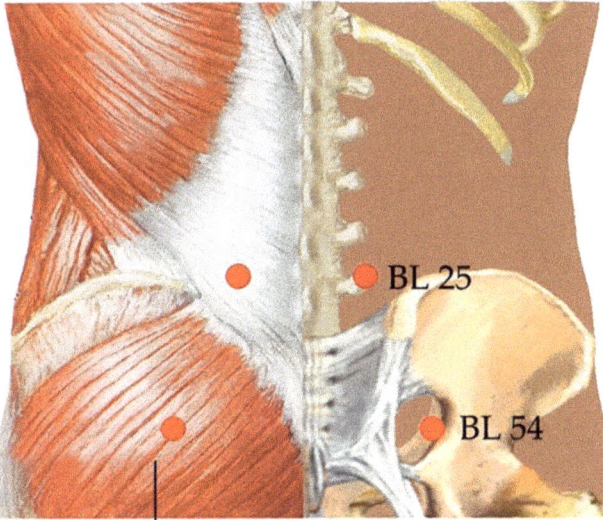

M. gluteus maximus

18. BL-27, BL-30 — Regulates the lower jiao, regulates the intestines and bladder

Indications	Weakness and pain of the lower back and knee, dysuria, constipation, irregular menstruation, hernia, spermatorrhea.

BL-27 — XiǎoChángShū

Position	On the lower back, 1.5 cun lateral to the lower border of the spinous process of the first sacral vertebra.
Acupoint Selection Skills	The point is located in the prone position, at the level with the inferior border of the spinous process of the first sacral vertebra, 1.5 cun lateral to the posterior middle line.
Regional Anatomy	The needle passes through the subcutaneous tissues and penetrates m. latissimus dorsi and m. sacrospinalis.
Acupuncture	Insert the needle perpendicularly 0.8~1.0 cun deep and stimulate until there is a sore and numbing sensation in the local area.

BL-30 — BáiHuánShū

Position	On the sacrum, 1.5 cun lateral to the middle of the sacral crest, at the level with the fourth posterior sacral foramen.
Acupoint Selection Skills	The point is located in the prone position, 1.5 cun lateral to the middle of the sacrum, at the level with the fourth posterior sacral foramen.
Regional Anatomy	The needle passes through the subcutaneous tissues and penetrates m. gluteus maximus.
Acupuncture	Insert the needle perpendicularly 1.0~1.5 cun deep and stimulate until there is a sore and numbing sensation in the local area radiating to the waist.

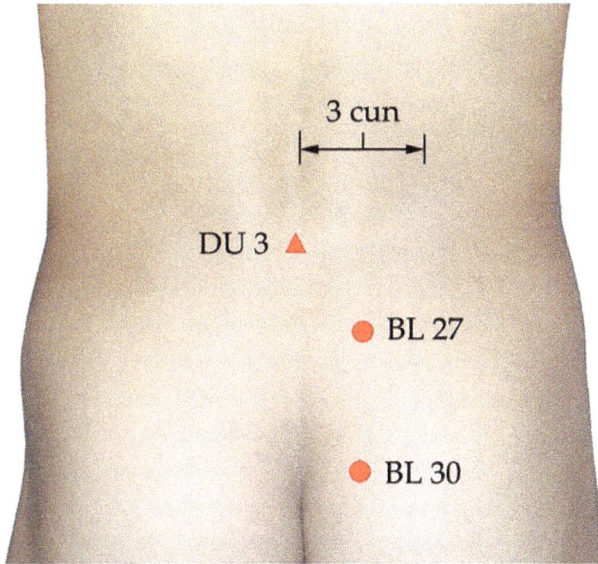

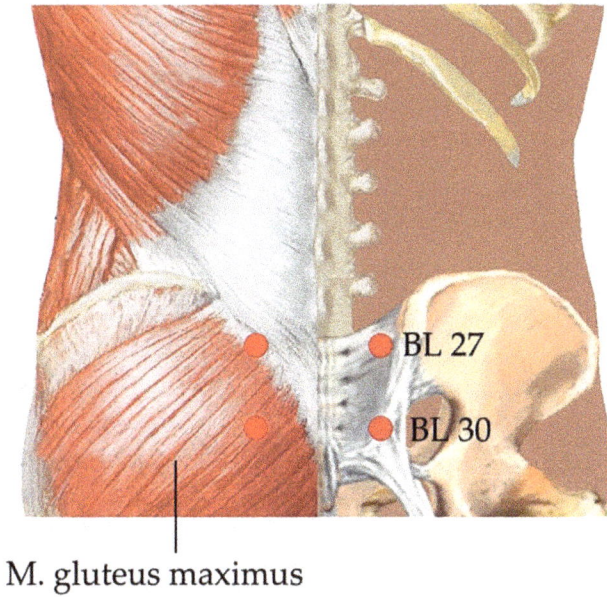

M. gluteus maximus

19. BL-32, BL-53 — Benefits original Qi, clears heat and resolves dampness, activates the channel and activates collaterals

Indications	Pain of the lumbosacral region, irregular menstruation, spermatorrhea, impotence, dysuria, constipation.

BL-32 — CìLiáo

Position	On the sacrum, medial and superior to the superior iliac spine, in the depression of the second posterior sacral foramen.
Regional Anatomy	The needle passes through the subcutaneous tissues and penetrates m. sacrospinalis.
Acupuncture	Insert the needle perpendicularly 0.8~1.0 cun deep and stimulate until there is a sore and numbing sensation in the local area radiating to the lower limbs.

BL-53 — BāoHuāng

Position	On the lower back, 3 cun lateral to the middle sacral crest, at the level with the second posterior sacral foramen.
Acupoint Selection Skills	The point is located in the prone position, 3 cun lateral to the second posterior sacral foramen.
Regional Anatomy	The needle passes through the subcutaneous tissues and penetrates m. gluteus medius.
Acupuncture	Insert the needle obliquely 0.8~1.0 cun deep and stimulate until there is a sore and numbing sensation in the local area radiating to the lower abdomen and hips.

3 cun

DU 3 ▲

BL 32 ●   ● BL 53

BL 32

BL 53

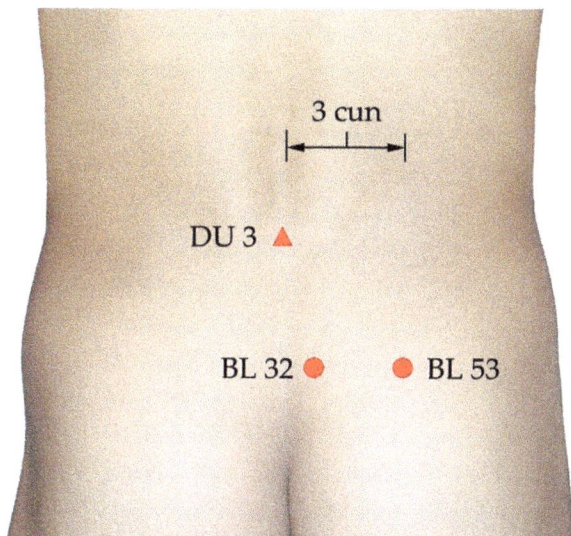

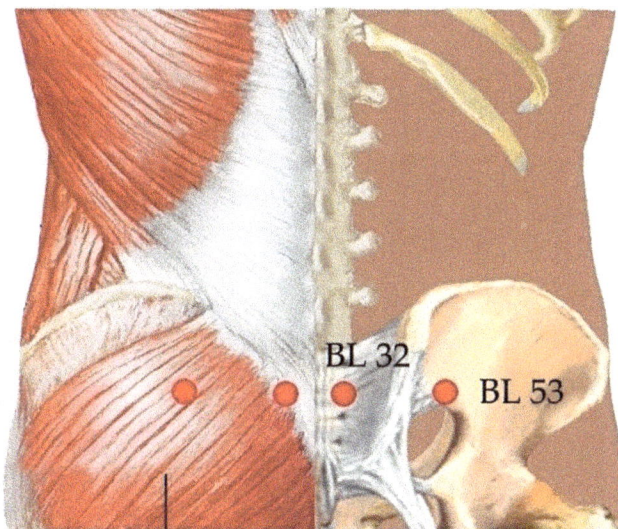

M. gluteus maximus

20. DU-2, DU-3 — Tonifies kidney and regulates menstruation, benefits the lumbar region and lower limbs

Indications	Pain of the lumbosacral region, blood in the stool, constipation, diarrhea, spermatorrhea, impotence, irregular menstruation.

DU-2 — YāoShū

Position	On the posterior midline in the hiatus of the sacrum.
Acupoint Selection Skills	The point is located in the prone position, on the posterior midline, at the level with the inferior border of the sacrum above the coccyx.
Regional Anatomy	The needle passes through the subcutaneous tissues and sacral canal and penetrates the sacral canal.
Acupuncture	Insert the needle perpendicularly 0.5~1.0 cun deep and stimulate until there is a sore and numbing sensation in the local area radiating to the lumbosacral region.

DU-3 — YāoYángGuān

Position	On the lumbar region, on the posterior midline, in the depression inferior to the spinous process of the fourth lumbar vertebra.
Acupoint Selection Skills	The point is located in the prone position, in the depression inferior to the spinous process of the fourth lumbar vertebra at the level with the crista iliaca.
Regional Anatomy	The needle passes through the subcutaneous tissues and supraspinal ligament and penetrates the interarcuate ligament.
Acupuncture	Insert the needle perpendicularly or obliquely 0.5~1.0 cun deep and stimulate until there is a sore and numbing sensation in the local area radiating to the lower limbs.

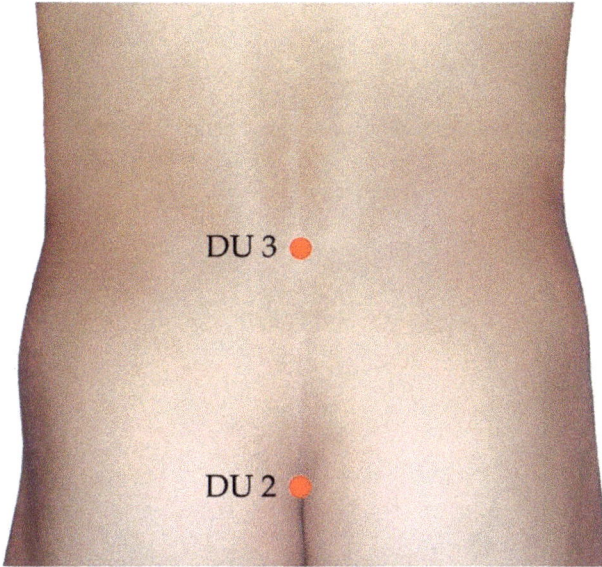

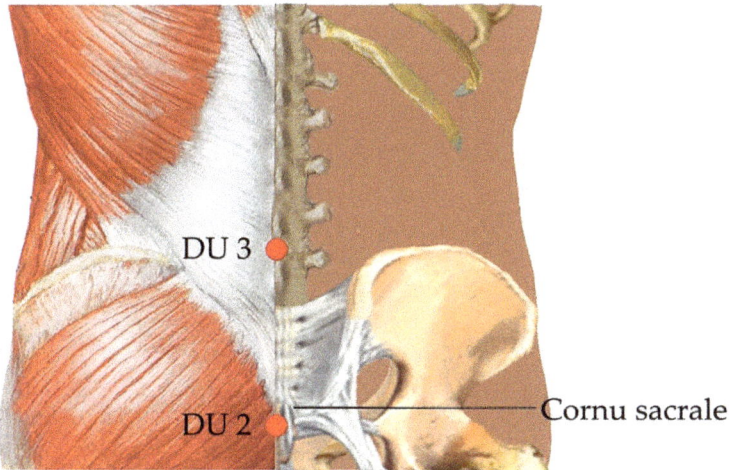

DU 3

DU 2

DU 3

DU 2

Cornu sacrale

CHAPTER 4

Extremities Combination Points

1. LI-15, SJ-14 — Dispels wind-dampness and alleviates pain, benefits the shoulder joint

Indications	Pain of the shoulder and arm, spasm of the arm and hand and hemiplegia.

LI-15 — JiānYú

Position	In the anterior and inferior aspect of the acromion, in the depression between the acromion and the greater tubercle of the humerus.
Acupoint Selection Skills	The point is located in the anterior depression on the shoulder joint when the arm is abducted at shoulder level. The point is also located approximately 2 cun posterior to the anterior end of the acromial end of the clavicle when the shoulder is adducted toward the body.
Regional Anatomy	The needle passes through the subcutaneous tissues and deeply towards HT 1 and reaches the plexus brachialis.
Acupuncture	Insert the needle perpendicularly 1.0~1.5 cun deep and stimulate until there is a sore and distending sensation in the local area.

SJ-14 — JiānLiáo

Position	On the shoulder, posterior to LI-15, when the arm is abducted, in the depression posterior and inferior to the acromion.
Acupoint Selection Skills	When the arm is abducted, there are two depression on the shoulder, the ante-rior depression is LI 15 and the posterior is SJ 14. Another method to locate SJ 14 is when the arm is adduct-ed, 2 cun inferior to the posterior and inferior border of the acromion end of the clavicle, between the acro-mion and the nodule of the humeral.
Regional Anatomy	The needle passes through the skin and subcutaneous fascia, penetrates m. deltoideus, enters m.teres minor and m. teres major.
Acupunc-ture	Insert the needle perpendicularly 1.0~1.5 cun deep and stimulate until there is a sore and distending sensation in the local area.

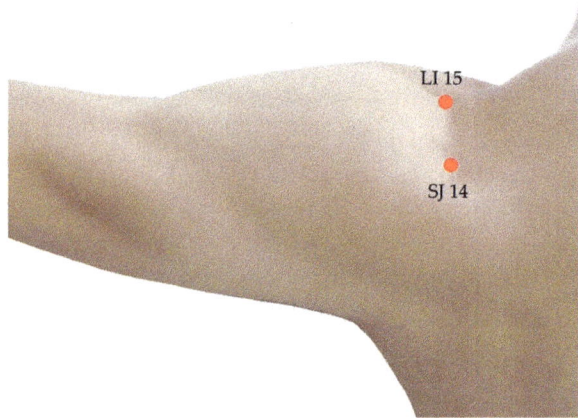

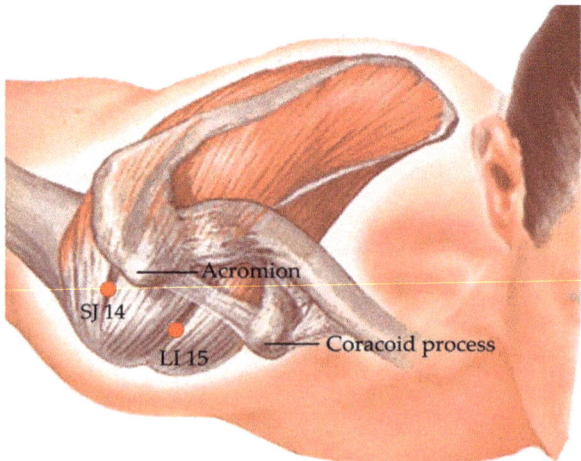

Acupuncture of Acupoint Combination

2. LU-5, PC-3 — Clears lung heat, activates the channel and relaxes the sinews, tonifies and nourishes the heart

Indications	Cough, asthma, hemoptysis, sore throat and chest distention, exanthemata, vomiting and diarrhea, spasmodic pain of the elbow and arm.

LU-5 — ChǎZé

Position	On the radial side of the tendon of m. biceps brachii at the level of the transverse cubital crease.
Acupoint Selection Skills	The point is located on the cubital crease when the elbow is slightly bent with the palm facing upward, on the radial side of the tendon of biceps brachii.
Regional Anatomy	The needle passes through the subcutaneous tissues and deep fascia, penetrates the m. brachioradialis.
Acupuncture	Insert the needle perpendicularly 0.5~1.0 cun deep and stimulate until there is a sore and numbing sensation in the local area with an electric sensation radiating to the forearm and palm.

PC-3 — QūZé

Position	On the transverse crease of the elbow, on the ulnar side of the tendon of m. biceps brachii.
Acupoint Selection Skills	The point is located when the arm is stretched forward with palm upward and the elbow flexed, on the transverse crease of the elbow.
Regional Anatomy	The needle passes through the skin and subcutaneous fascia, pierces the anterior cubital fascia between v. basilica and intermedian cubital vein, reaches the trunk of n. medianus and m. brachialis at the medial side of the brachial artery.
Acupuncture	Insert the needle perpendicularly 0.5~1.0 cun deep and stimulate until there is a numbing and distending sensation in the local area radiating to the the middle finger.

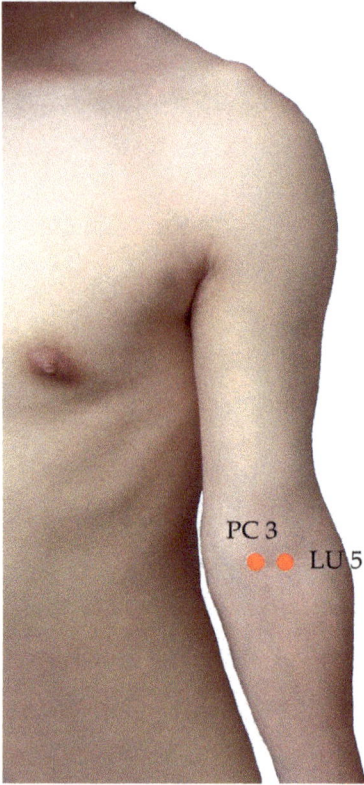

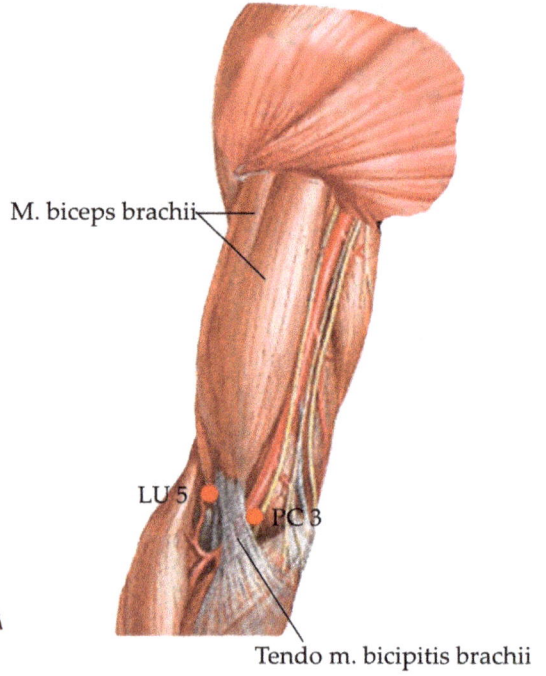

PC 3

LU 5

M. biceps brachii

LU 5

PC 3

Tendo m. bicipitis brachii

3. LI-11, LI-4 — Relieves the surface and clears heat, activates collaterals to relieve pain

Indications	Headache, nasal obstruction, toothache, sore throat, deviation of the eye and mouth, cough and asthma, abdominal pain, dysentery, dysmenorrhea, paralysis of the upper limb, vomiting, diarrhea, urticaria, cutaneous pruritus.

LI-11 — QūChí

Position	In the depression of the radial side of the transverse cubital crease when elbow flexed.
Acupoint Selection Skills	The point is located when the elbow is flexed in the depression at the lateral end of the transverse cubital crease, midway between LU 5 and the lateral epicondyle of the humerus.
Regional Anatomy	The needle passes through the subcutaneous tissues, enters the m. extensor carpi radialis longus and m. extensor carpi radialis brevis, reaches the m. brachioradialis, penetrates through the truncus n. radialis and reaches the m. brachialis.
Acupuncture	Insert the needle perpendicularly 1.0~1.5 cun deep and stimulate until there is a sore and numbing sensation in the local area radiating to the shoulder or the fingers.

LI-4 — HéGǎ

Position	On the dorsum of the hand, between the first and second metacarpal bones, on the radial side of the middle of the second metacarpal bone.
Acupoint Selection Skills	The point is located in the web between the index finger and the thumb when the thumb and index are stretched apart, at the middle point of the first metacarpal bone. Another method is by locating the highest part of the m. adductor pollicis when the thumb and index finger are pressed together.
Regional Anatomy	The needle passes through the subcutaneous tissues, enters the m. interossedorsales (1st), and penetrates the m. adductor pollicis from the medial side of the dorsal venous network and deep palmar artery.
Acupuncture	Insert the needle perpendicularly 0.5~1.0 cun deep and stimulte until there is a sore and numbing sensation in the local area radiating to the end of the fingers.

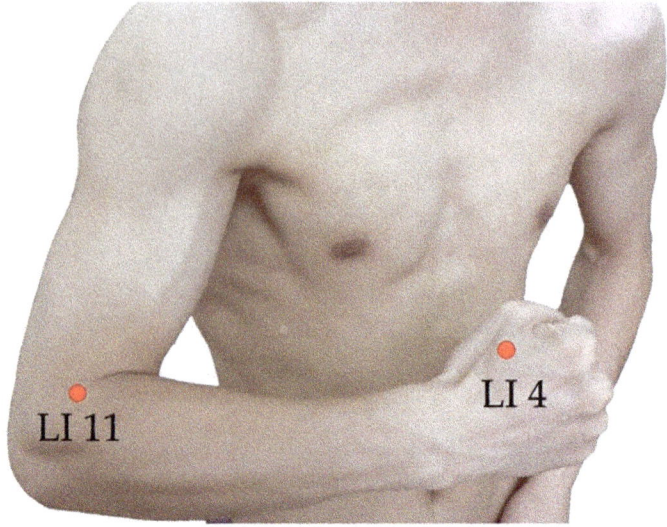

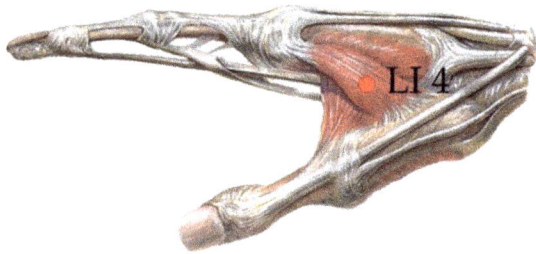

LI 11

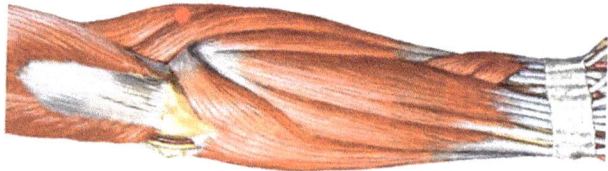

4. LI-5, SJ-4, SI-5 — Expels wind and clears heat, activates the channel and alleviates pain

Indications	Redness, swelling and pain of the eye, pain in the wrist, febrile disease.

LI-5 — YángXī

Position	On the dorsal side of the wrist, in the depression between the tendons of m. extensor pollicis longus and m. extensor pollicis brevis.
Acupoint Selection Skills	The point is located in the depression between the tendons of m. extensor pol-licis longus and brevis on the dorsal side of the wrist when the thumb is pointing upward.
Regional Anatomy	The needle passes through this ligament, runs between the tendons of m. extensor pollicis longus and m. extensor pollicis brevis, and arrives at the dorsal side of the tendon of m. extensor carpi radialis longus.
Acupuncture	Insert the needle perpendicularly 0.5~0.8 cun deep and stimulate until there is a sore and numbing sensation in the local area.

SJ-4 — YángChí

Position	On the dorsum aspect of the transverse wrist crease, in the depression on the ulnar side of the tendon of m. extensor digitorumcommunis.
Acupoint Selection Skills	On the ulnar side of the dorsum aspect of the wrist, be-tween the tendon of musculus extensor digitorumcom-munis and extesnordigitiquintiproprius.
Regional Anatomy	The needle passes through the skin and subcutaneous fascia, pierces the deep fascia, runs between m. extensor digitiminimiandtendo m. extensor digitorum, and reach-es the surface of Os tri-quetrum. m. extensor digitiminim-iand m. extensor digitorum.
Acupuncture	Insert the needle perpendicularly 0.3~0.5 cun deep and stimulate until there is a sore and distending sensation in the local area radiating to the middle finger.

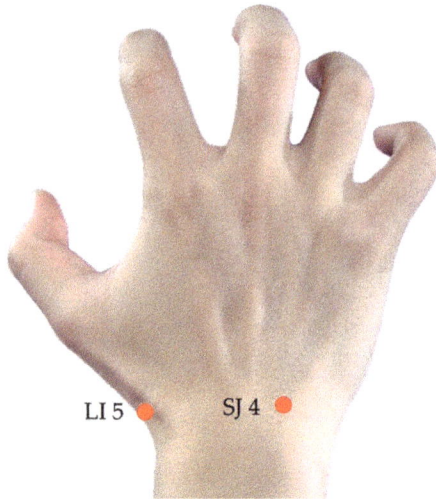

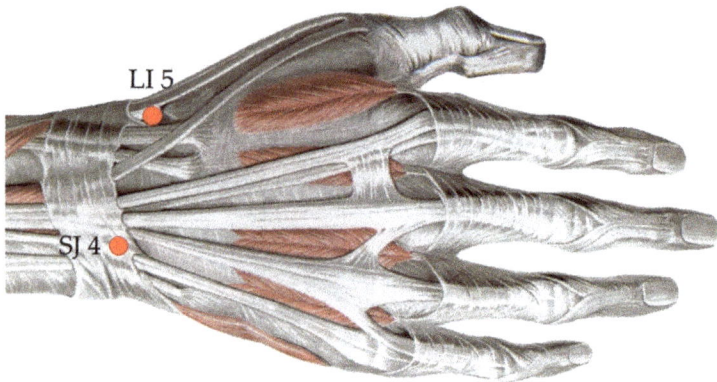

SI-5 — YángGǎ

Position	On the ulnar side of the wrist, in the depression between the styloid process of the ulna and the triangular bone.
Acupoint Selection Skills	The point is located proximal to the triangular bone when the palm is facing down, proximal to SI-4.
Regional Anatomy	The needle passes through the skin and subcutaneous tissue, penetrates ligamentpi-sometacarpeum and reaches the periost of the unciform bone.
Acupuncture	Insert the needle perpendicularly 0.3~0.5 cun deep and stimulate until there is a sore and numbing sensation in the local area radiating in the wrist.

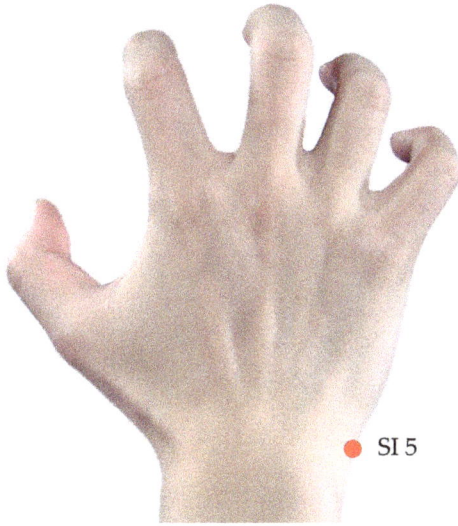

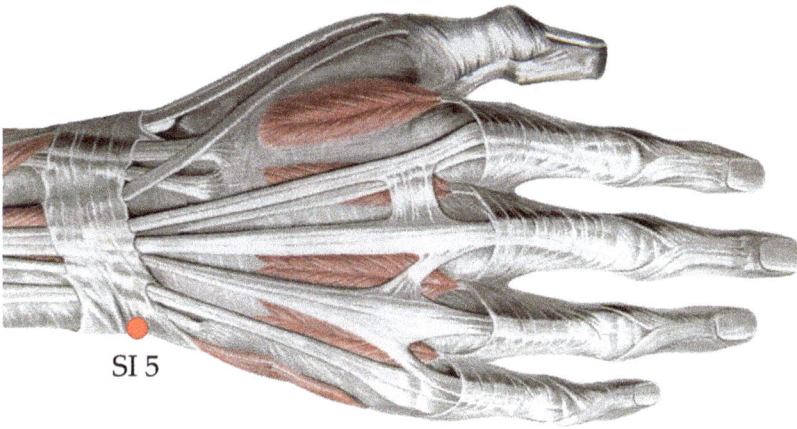

SI 5

SI 5

5. PC-6, PC-4 — Regulates Qi and alleviates pain, descends rebellious Qi and regulates stomach, calms the spirit

Indications	Cardiac pain, palpitation and insomnia, stomach ache, vomiting and hiccough, elbow and arm contracture pain.

PC-6 — NèiGuān

Position	On the palmar aspect of the forearm, 2 cun superior to the transverse crease of the wrist, be-tween the tendon of m.palmaris longus and m. flexor carpi radialis.
Acupoint Selection Skills	The point is located on the forearm with the palm upward and the wrist is slightly flexed, 2 cun superior to the midpoint of the transverse crease of the wrist, on the line connecting PC-3 to PC-7, between the tendon of m.palmaris longus and m. flexor carpi radialis.
Regional Anatomy	The needle passes through the skin and subcutaneous fascia, pierces the deep brachial fascia, reaches m. flexor digitorumsuperficialis between m. palmaris longus and m. flexor carpi radialis, en-ters m. flexor digitorumprofundus and m. pronator quadratus.
Acupuncture	Insert the needle perpendicularly 0.5~1.5 cun deep and stimulate until there is a sore and numbing sensation in the local area with an electric sensation radiating to the finger tip.

PC-4 — XìMén

Position	On the palmar side of the forearm, 5 cun superior to the transverse crease of the wrist, between the tendon of m.palmaris longus and m. flexor carpi radialis.
Acupoint Selection Skills	The point is located when the arm is stretched forward with palm upward and the elbow flexed, 5 cun above the midpoint of the transverse crease of the wrist, on the line connecting PC-3 to PC-7, between the tendon of m.palmaris longus and m. flexor carpi radialis.

Regional Anatomy	The needle passes through the skin and subcutaneous fascia, penetrates the deep bra-chial fascia and the muscular layer, and reaches membrane ainterosseaantebra-chii.
Acupuncture	Insert the needle perpendicularly 0.5~0.8 cun deep and stimulate until there is a sore and numbing sensation in the local area radiating to the finger tip.

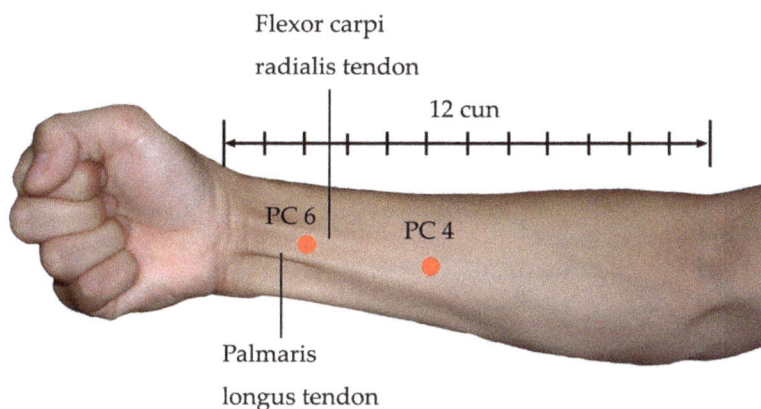

Flexor carpi radialis tendon

12 cun

PC 6

PC 4

Palmaris longus tendon

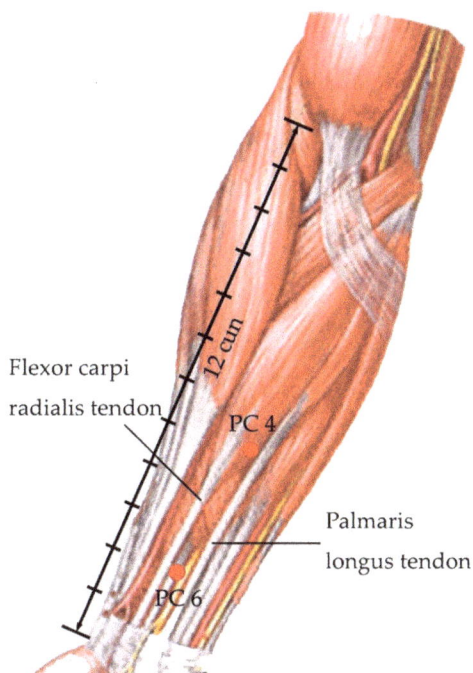

Flexor carpi radialis tendon

12 cun

PC 4

Palmaris longus tendon

PC 6

6. PC 6, HT-7, PC-7 — Unbinds the chest and regulates Qi, regulates heart and calms the spirit

Indications	Cardiac pain and palpitation, insomnia, irritability, mental depression.

PC-6 — NèiGuān

Position	On the palmar aspect of the forearm, 2 cun superior to the transverse crease of the wrist, be-tween the tendon of m.palmaris longus and m. flexor carpi radialis.
Acupoint Selection Skills	The point is located on the forearm with the palm upward and the wrist is slightly flexed, 2 cun superior to the midpoint of the transverse crease of the wrist, on the line connecting PC-3 to PC-7, between the tendon of m.palmaris longus and m. flexor carpi radialis.
Regional Anatomy	The needle passes through the skin and subcutaneous fascia, pierces the deep brachial fascia, reaches m. flexor digitorumsuperficialis between m. palmaris longus and m. flexor carpi radialis, en-ters m. flexor digitorumprofundus and m. pronator quadratus.
Acupuncture	Insert the needle perpendicularly 0.5~1.5 cun deep and stimulate until there is a sore and numbing sensation in the local area with an electric sensation radiating to the finger tip.

HT-7 — ShénMén

Position	On the radial side of the tendon m. flexor carpi ulnaris of the transverse wrist crease.
Acupoint Selection Skills	The point is located on the radial side of the tendon m. flexor carpi ulnaris, on the transverse wrist crease when the palm is facing upwards.

Regional Anatomy	The needle passes through the skin and subcutis, penetrates the deep fascia of the arm from the radial border of m. flexor carpi ulnaris, reaches the head of the ulna from the medial side of n. ulnaris and the ulnar artery and vein.
Acupuncture	Insert the needle perpendicularly 0.3~0.5 cun deep and stimulates until there is a sore and numbing sensation in the local area.

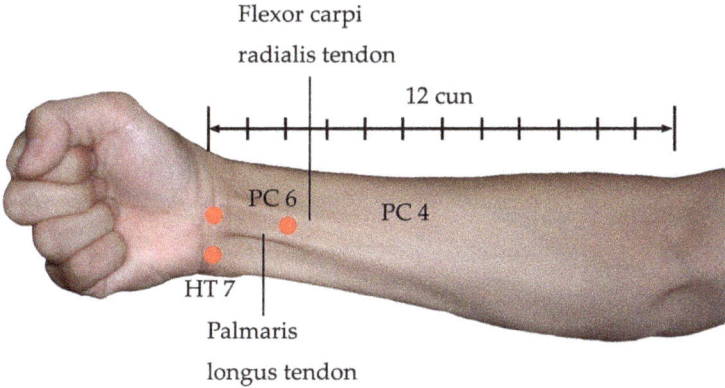

Flexor carpi radialis tendon

12 cun

PC 6

PC 4

HT 7

Palmaris longus tendon

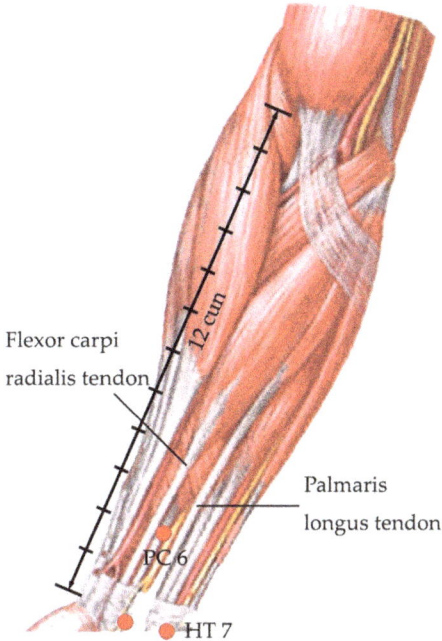

Flexor carpi radialis tendon

12 cun

Palmaris longus tendon

PC 6

HT 7

PC-7 — DàLíng

Position	On the palmar side of the forearm, in the middle of the transverse crease of the wrist, between the tendon of m.palmaris longus and m. flexor carpi radialis.
Acupoint Selection Skills	The point is located when the arm is stretched forward with palm upward and the elbow flexed, in the midpoint of the transverse crease of the wrist, between the tendon of m.palmaris lon-gus and m. flexor carpi radialis.
Regional Anatomy	The needle passes through the skin and subcutaneous fascia, penetrates the deep bra-chial fascia and reaches intercarpal joint capsule.
Acupuncture	Insert the needle perpendicularly 0.3~0.5 cun deep and stimulate until there is a sore and numbing sensation in the local area with an electric sensation radiating to the finger tip.

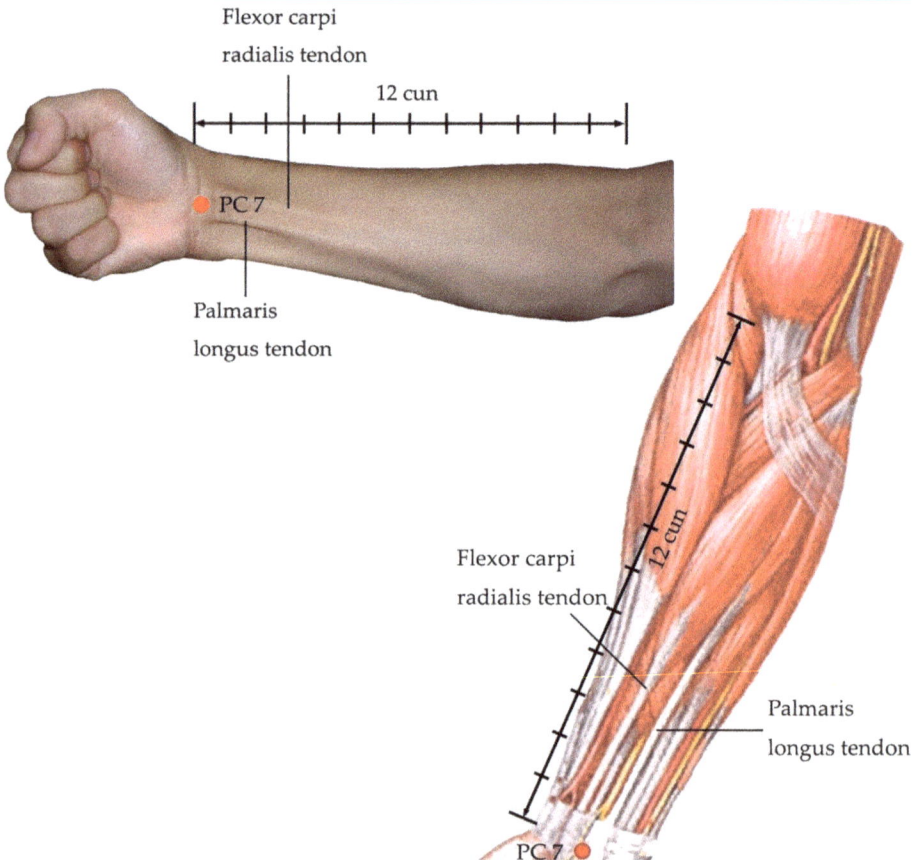

Flexor carpi radialis tendon

12 cun

PC 7

Palmaris longus tendon

Flexor carpi radialis tendon

12 cun

Palmaris longus tendon

PC 7

7. LU-7, LU-9 — Releases the exterior and expels wind, alleviates cough and transforms phlegm

Indications	Cough, asthma, hemoptysis, headache, sore throat, neck stiffness.

LU-7 — LièQuē

Position	On the radial side of the forearm, 1.5 cun proximal the transverse crease of the wrist, superior to the styloid process of the radius and between tendons of m. brachioradialis and m. abductor pollicis longus.
Acupoint Selection Skills	The point is located by crossing the webs of the thumbs and placing the index finger on the styloid process of the radius of the other hand. The point located under the tip of the index finger in the depression of the styloid process. Another locating method is by first locating LI-5, LU-7 is 1.5 cundistal to LI-5.
Regional Anatomy	The needle passes through the subcutaneous tissues and abductor pollicis longus tendon and penetrates m. pronator quadratus.
Acupuncture	Insert the needle obliquely upward 0.2~0.3 cun deep and stimulate until there is a sore, heavy and numbing sensation in the local area.

LU-9 — TàiYuān

Position	On the radial end of the wrist crease, where the radial pulse is palpable.
Acupoint Selection Skills	The point is located when the palm is facing upwards, on the transverse wrist crease where the radial pulse is palpable.
Regional Anatomy	The needle passes through the subcutaneous tissues and goes between the v. cephalica and the superficial branch of a. radialis, penetrates through the antebrachial fascia, runs from the lateral side of the a. radialis and v. radialis, and arrives at the periost of the radius between the tendons of m. abductor pollicis longus and m. flexor carpi radialis.
Acupuncture	Insert the needle perpendicularly 0.2~0.3 cun deep and stimulate until there is a numbing and distending sensation in the local area. Avoid puncturing the radial artery.

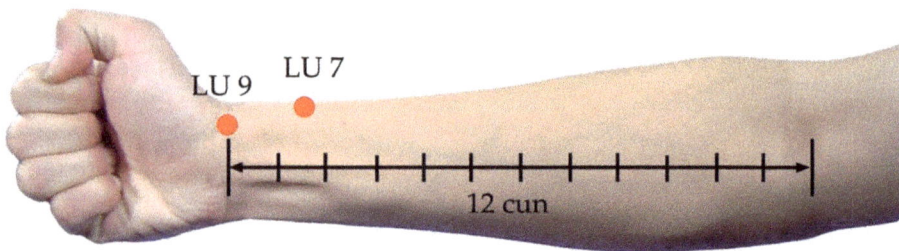

LU 9   LU 7

12 cun

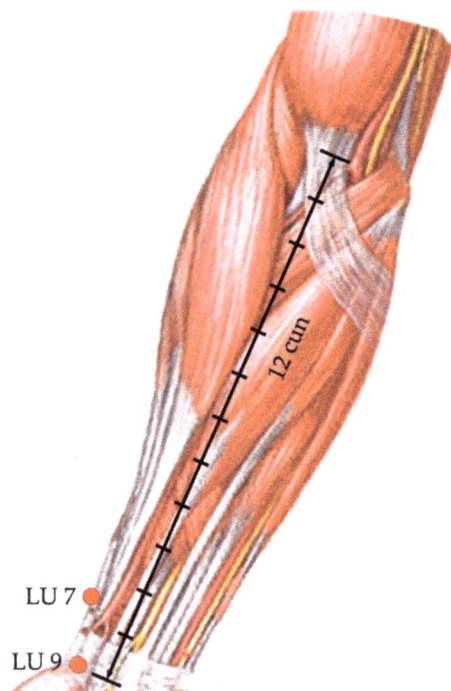

LU 7

LU 9

12 cun

8. LI-13, LI-14 — Expels wind and activates the channel, regulates Qi and transforms phlegm

Indications	Swelling and pain of the arm and paralysis of the upper limb, malaria, scrofula.

LI-13 — ShǒuWǔLǐ

Position	On the lateral aspect of the humerus, 3 cun proximal to LI-11 on the line connecting LI-11 andLI-15.
Acupoint Selection Skills	The point is located when the elbow is flexed, 3 cun proximal to LI-11 on the line connecting LI-11 and LI-15.
Regional Anatomy	The needle passes through the subcutaneous tissues and penetrates the m. brachialis.
Acupuncture	Insert the needle perpendicularly 0.5~1.0 cun deep and stimulate until there is a sore and numbing sensation in the local area.

LI-14 — BìNào

Position	On the lateral side of the upper arm, 7 cun proximal to LI -11, in the depression formed by the distal insertion of the m.deltoideus and m. brachialis.
Regional Anatomy	The needle passes through the skin and subcutaneous tissue and penetrates the mid-point of the m. deltoideus.
Acupuncture	Insert the needle perpendicularly 0.5~1.0 cun deep and stimulate until there is a sore and numbing sensation in the local area.

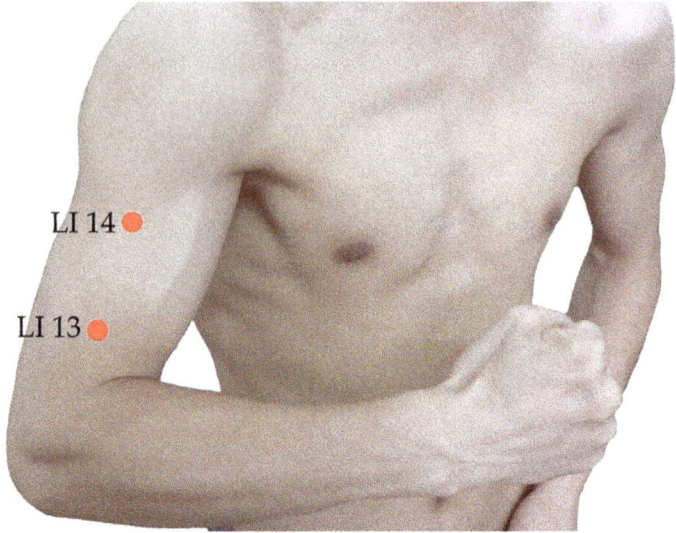

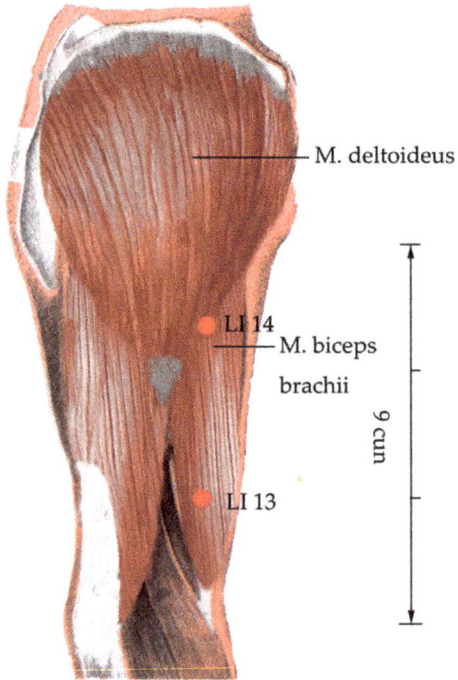

M. deltoideus

LI 14 — M. biceps
brachii

9 cun

LI 13

9. LU-10, SJ-2 — Descends lung Qi and relieves sore-throat, relieves the surface and clears heat

Indications	Swelling and sore throat, headache, malaria

LU-10 — YúJì

Position	In the depression proximal to the metacarpophalange-al joint, on the radial side of the midpoint of the meta-carpal bone, at the junction of the red and white skin.
Acupoint Selection Skills	The point is located when the hand is in a loose fist with the palm facing up-wards, at the juncture of the red and white skin in the middle of the first metacarpal bone.
Regional Anatomy	The needle passes through the subcutaneous tissues and m. abductor pollicis brevis, and penetrates m. opponenspollicis and m. flexor pollicis brevis.
Acupuncture	Insert the needle perpendicularly 0.3~0.5 cun deep and stimulate until there is a distending sensation in the local area.

SJ-2 — YèMén

Position	On the dorsum aspect of the hand, proximal to the margin of the web between the fourth and fifth finger, at the junction of the red and white skin.
Acupoint Selection Skills	The point is located when the hand makes a loose fist and the palm is facing downwards, at the edge of the web between the fourth and fifth finger, at the junction of the red and white skin.
Regional Anatomy	The needle passes through the skin and subcutaneous tissue, penetrates the inter-tendinous connection formed by the 3rd and 4th tendons of m. extensor digitorum and reaches m. interos-seidorsales and the ulnar nerve.
Acupuncture	Insert the needle perpendicularly 0.3~0.5 cun deep and stimulate until there is a sore and distending sensation in the local area radiating to the dorsum of the hand.

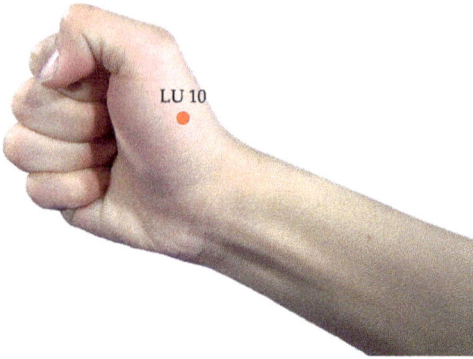

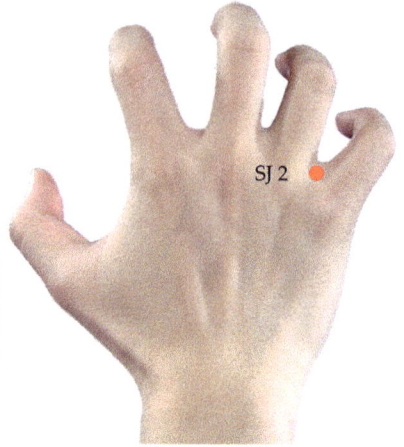

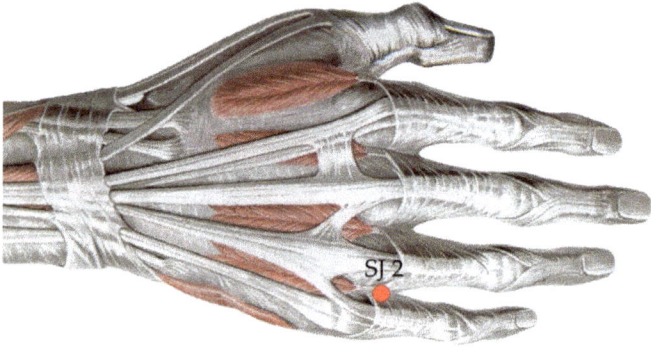

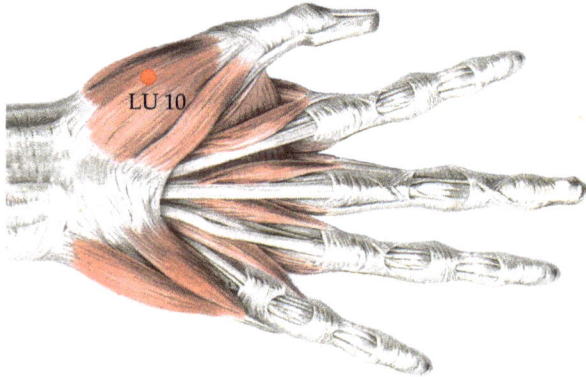

Acupuncture of Acupoint Combination

10. HT-6, SI-3 — Benefits the head and eyes, calms spirit

Indications	Cardiac pain, night sweat, malaria, redness, swelling and pain of the eye, tinnitus.

HT-6 — YīnXì

Position	On the palmar side of the forearm, on the line connecting HT-7 to HT-3, 0.5 cun proximal to HT-7.
Acupoint Selection Skills	The point is located on the radial side of the tendon m. flexor carpi ulnaris, 0.5 cun proximal to the transverse wrist crease when the palm is facing upwards.
Regional Anatomy	The needle passes the skin and subcutaneous fascia, penetrates the deep fascia of arm, and reaches the region between n. ulnaris and the ulnar artery and vein from the radial border of m. flexor carpi ulnaris.
Acupuncture	Insert the needle perpendicularly 0.3~0.5 cun deep and stimulate until there is a sore and numbing sensation in the local area radiating down the channel and reaching the ring or little finger or reach-ing the axilla, head and chest.

SI-3 — HòuXī

Position	On the ulnar side of the hand, proximal to the fifth metacarpophalangeal joint, at the end of the transverse crease, at the the junction of the red and white skin side.
Acupoint Selection Skills	The point is located on the ulnar side of the hand, at the junction of the red and white skin, proximal to the fifth metacarpophalangeal joint when the fist is loose.
Regional Anatomy	The needle passes through the skin and subcutaneous tissue, enters m. abductor digit-iminimi, and reaches the region between m. flexor digitiminimi brevis manus and the 5th metacarpal bone.
Acupuncture	Insert the needle perpendicularly towards LI-4 0.5~0.8 cun deep and stimulate until there is a sore and numbing sensation in the local area, spreading in the palm.

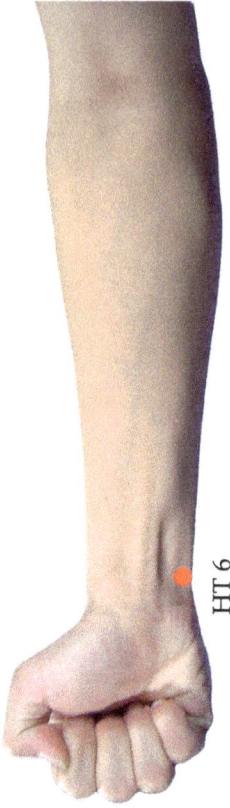

HT 6

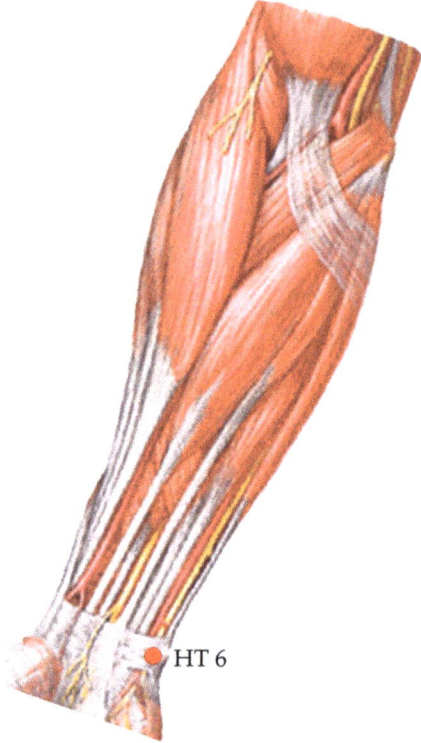

HT 6

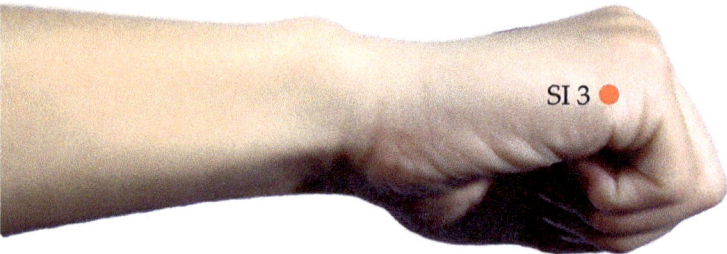

SI 3

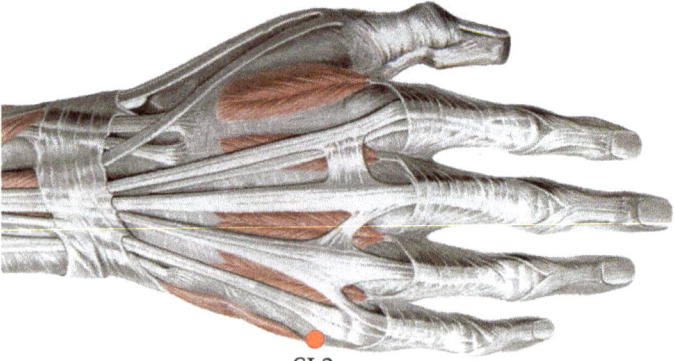

SI 3

11. BL-63, BL-61 — Relaxes sinews and activates channel, calms spirit

Indications	Headache, infantile convulsion, weakness of the lower extremities and pain of the heel, foot sprain.

BL-63 — JīnMén

Position	On the lateral side of the foot, inferior to the anterior border of the external malleolus, lateral to the lower border of the cuboid bone.
Acupoint Selection Skills	The point is located in the supine position, 0.5 cun anterior and inferior to BL-62.
Regional Anatomy	The needle passes through the subcutaneous tissues and penetratesperiost of calcaneus.
Acupuncture	Insert the needle perpendicularly 0.3~0.5 cun deep and stimulate until there is a sore and numbing sensation in the local area spreading to the dorsum pedis.

BL-61 — PúCān

Position	On the lateral side of the foot, posterior and inferior to the external malleolus, inferior to BL 60, lateral to the calcaneum at the junction of the red and white skin.
Acupoint Selection Skills	The point is located in the sitting position with the foot resting on the ground, posterior and inferior to the external malleolus, inferior to BL-60, lateral to the calcaneum at the junction of the red and white skin.
Regional Anatomy	The needle passes through the subcutaneous tissues and penetratescalcaneo fibular ligament.
Acupuncture	Insert the needle perpendicularly 0.3~0.5 cun deep and stimulate until there is a sore and numbing sensation in the local area.

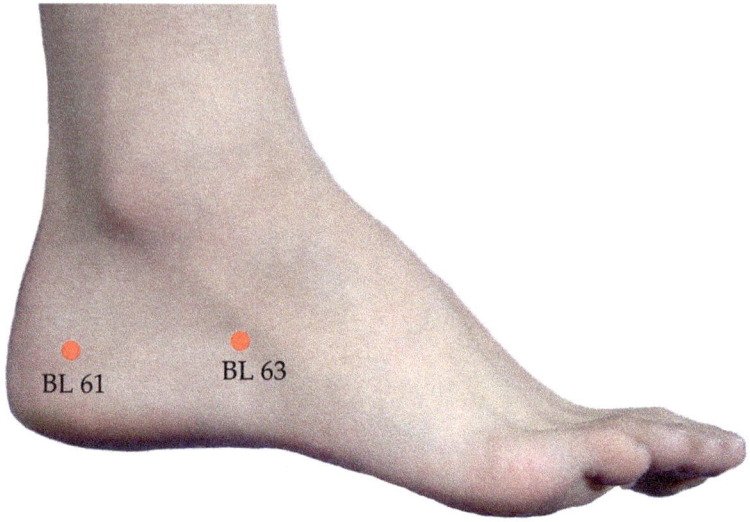

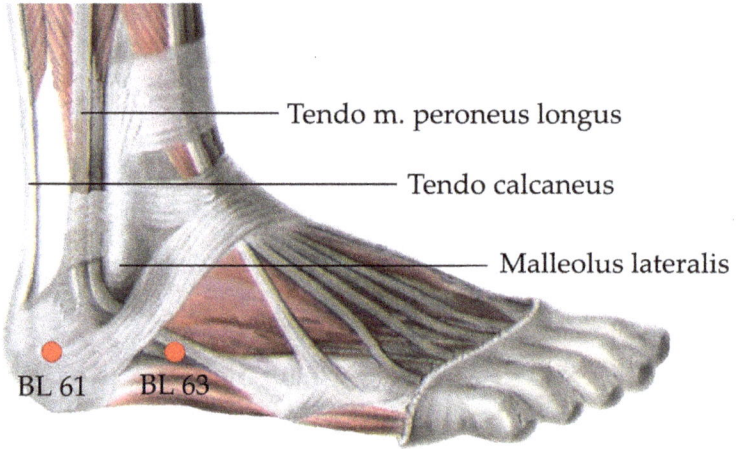

Tendo m. peroneus longus

Tendo calcaneus

Malleolus lateralis

12. GB-30, BL-36 — Benefits the lumbar region and lower limbs, dispels wind and damp

Indications	Lumbar pain, weakness and numbness of the lower back and limbs, sciatica, swelling and pain of the knee and ankle, hemiplegia.

GB-30 — HuánTiào

Position	On the lateral aspect of the body, when the thigh is flexed, at the junction of the lateral 1/3 and medial 2/3 of the line connecting the greater trochanter and the hiatus of the sacrum.
Acupoint Selection Skills	The point is located in the lateral position when the thigh is flexed and the leg is bent, first locate the greater trochanter and the hiatus of the sacrum, at the lateral 1/3 and medial 2/3 of the line connecting the greater trochanter and hiatus of the sacrum.
Regional Anatomy	The needle passes through the subcutaneous tissues and penetrates the m. obturatorius internus.
Acupuncture	Insert the needle obliquely downwards 2.0~3.0 cun deep and stimulate until there is a sore and numbing sensation in the local area radiating to the lower limbs.

BL-36 — ChéngFú

Position	On the posterior side of the thigh, in the middle of the transverse gluteal fold.
Regional Anatomy	The needle passes through the subcutaneous tissues and penetrates the trunk of n. ischiadicus.
Acupuncture	Insert the needle perpendicularly 1.5~2.5 cun deep and stimulate until there is a sore and numbing sensation in the local area radiating to the foot.

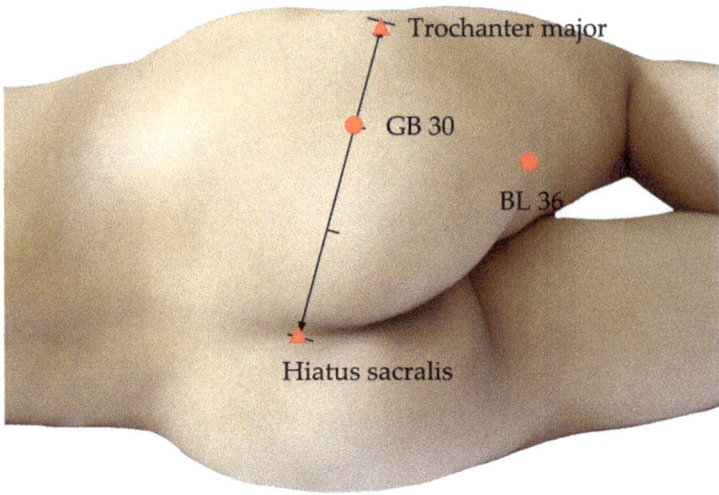

Trochanter major

GB 30

BL 36

Hiatus sacralis

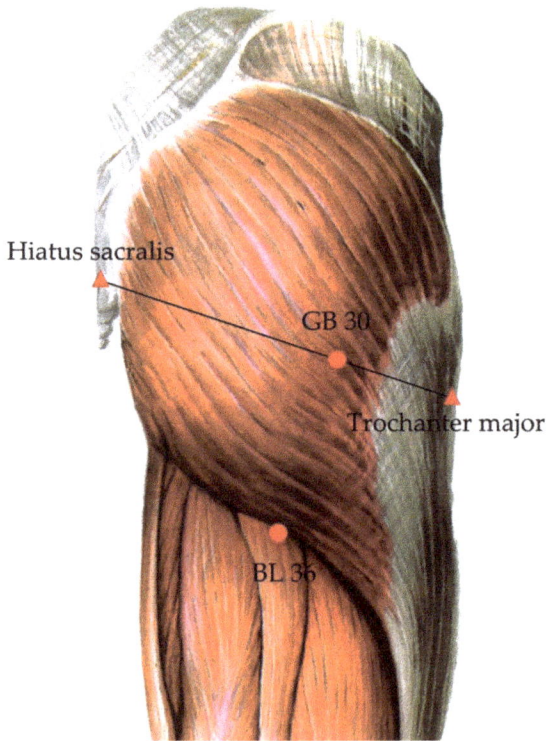

Hiatus sacralis

GB 30

Trochanter major

BL 36

13. ST-33, GB-31 — Dispels wind and damp, regulates Qi and blood

Indications	Coldness, pain and paralysis of the leg and knee, weakness and numbness of the lower limbs, itching of the whole body.

ST-33 — YīnShì

Position	On the anterior aspect of the thigh, on the line connecting the anterior superior iliac spine and the lateral end of the patella, 3 cun proximal to the patella.
Acupoint Selection Skills	The point is located in the sitting position when the knee is flexed, the point is four finger-width above lateral superior border of the patella.
Regional Anatomy	The needle passes through the subcutaneous tissues and penetrates the m. vastus lat-eralis.
Acupuncture	Insert the needle perpendicularly 1.0~1.5 cun deep and stimulate until there is a sore and numbing sensation in the local area radiating to the knee.

GB-31 — FēngShì

Position	On the midline of the lateral aspect of the thigh, 7 cun proximal to the transverse popliteal crease, at the level with the tip of the middle finger placed naturally on the thigh, between m. vastus lateralis and m. biceps femoris.
Acupoint Selection Skills	The point is located in the standing position with the hand resting on the side of the body, at the level with the tip of the middle finger placed naturally on the thigh.
Regional Anatomy	The needle passes through the subcutaneous tissues and penetrates the m. vastus in-termedius.
Acupuncture	Insert the needle perpendicularly 1.5~2.5 cun deep and stimulate until there is a sore and numbing sensation in the local area.

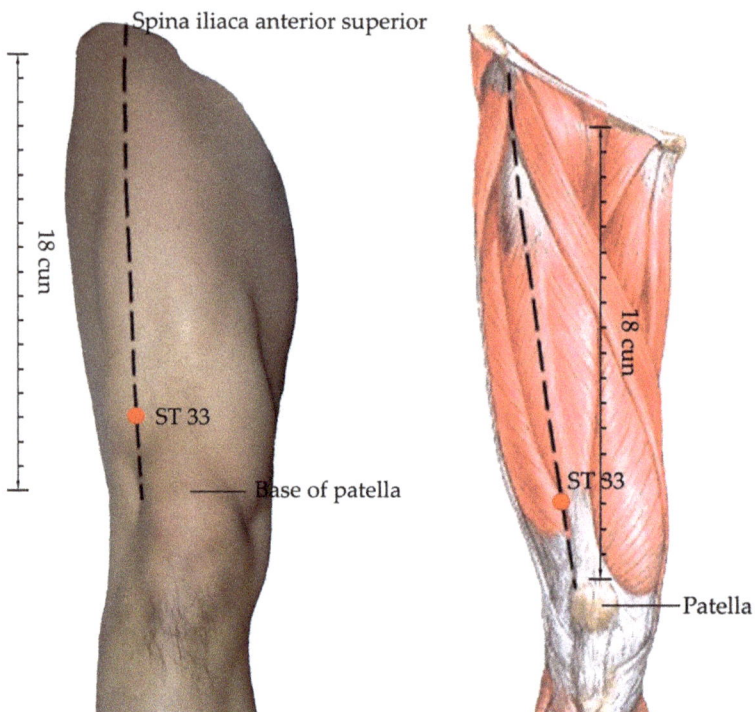

Spina iliaca anterior superior

18 cun

ST 33

Base of patella

18 cun

ST 33

Patella

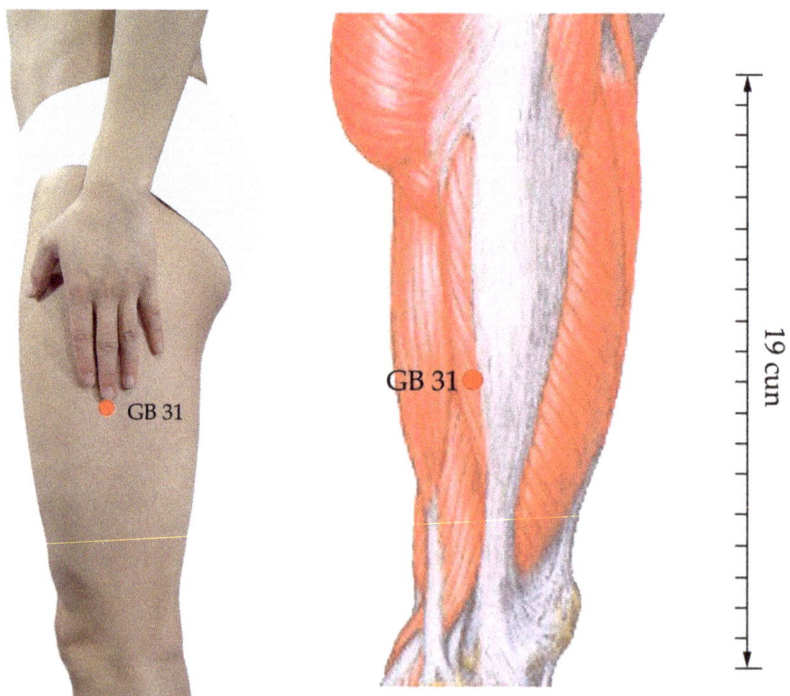

GB 31

GB 31

19 cun

14. GB-34, ST-36 — Invigorates the spleen and harmonizes the stomach, supports the correct Qi and nourish the original Qi, activates the channel and alleviates pain.

Indications	Headache, stomach ache, vomiting, abdominal distention, tinnitus, pain of the eye, pain and distention in the hypochondrium, cough and asthma, jaundice enuresis, weakness and numbness of the lower limbs, hemiplegia.

GB-34 — YángLíngQuán

Position	The point is located in the sitting position with the knee bent at 90° or in the supine position, in the depression anterior and inferior to the head of the fibula.
Regional Anatomy	The needle passes through the subcutaneous tissues and penetrates the m. peroneus brevis.
Acupuncture	Insert the needle perpendicularly towards SP 9 1.0~1.5 cun deep and stimulate until there is a sore and numbing sensation in the local area radiating downwards.

ST-36 — ZúSānLǐ

Position	On the anterior aspect of the lower leg, 3 cun distal to ST 35, one finger width lateral from the anterior ridge of the tibia.
Acupoint Selection Skills	① The point is located in the sitting position when the knee is bent, 3 cun to ST-35, one finger width lateral to the anterior ridge of the tibia. ② The point is located in the sitting position when the knee is bent, 1 cun below the outer inferior margin of tibial trochanter.
Regional Anatomy	The needle passes through the subcutaneous tissues and penetrates m. tibialis anterior and m. extensor hallucis longus.
Acupuncture	Insert the needle perpendicularly 0.5~1.5 cun deep and stimulate until there is a sensation radiating to the ankle and dorsum of the foot and toes.

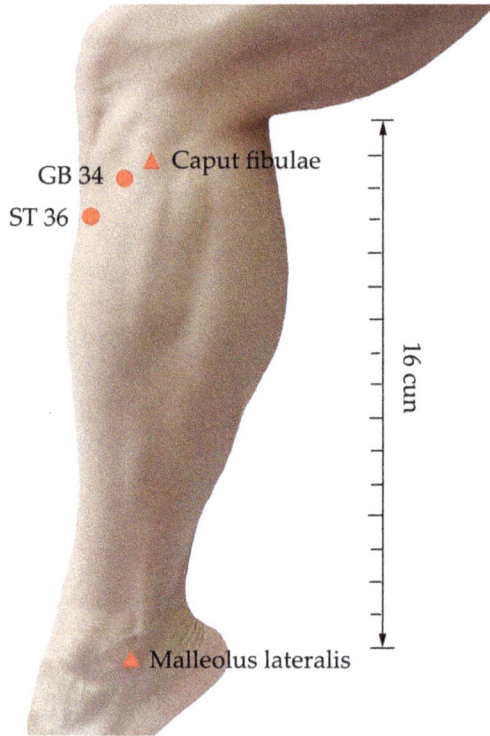

GB 34
ST 36
Caput fibulae
16 cun
Malleolus lateralis

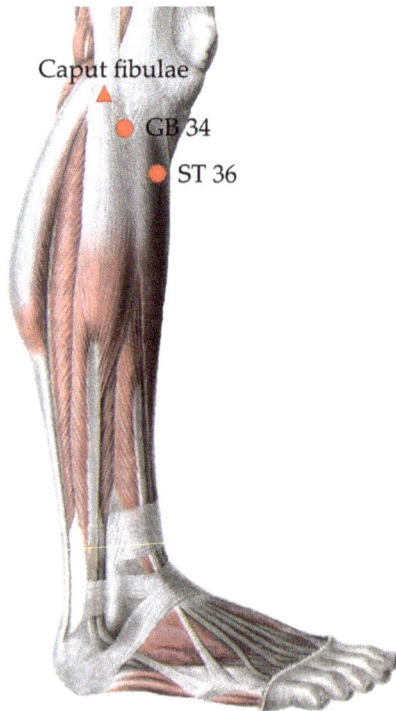

Caput fibulae
GB 34
ST 36

15. GB-34, LI-11 — Clears heat and expels wind, activates the channel and alleviates pain

Indications	Headache, tinnitus, asthma and cough, weakness and numbness of the lower extremities and hemiplegia.

GB-34 — YángLíngQuán

Position	The point is located in the sitting position with the knee bent at 90° or in the supine position, in the depression anterior and inferior to the head of the fibula.
Regional Anatomy	The needle passes through the subcutaneous tissues and penetrates the m. peroneus brevis.
Acupuncture	Insert the needle perpendicularly towards SP 9 1.0~1.5 cun deep and stimulate until there is a sore and numbing sensation in the local area radiating downwards.

LI-11 — QūChí

Position	In the depression of the radial side of the transverse cubital crease when elbow flexed.
Acupoint Selection Skills	The point is located when the elbow is flexed in the depression at the lateral end of the transverse cubital crease, midway between LU-5 and the lateral epicondyle of the humerus.
Regional Anatomy	The needle passes through the subcutaneous tissues, enters the m. extensor carpi radialis longus and m. extensor carpi radialis brevis, reaches the m. brachioradialis, penetrates through the truncus n. radialis and reaches the m. brachialis.
Acupuncture	Insert the needle perpendicularly 1.0~2.0 cun deep and stimulate until there is a sore and numbing sensation in the local area radiating to the shoulder or the fingers.

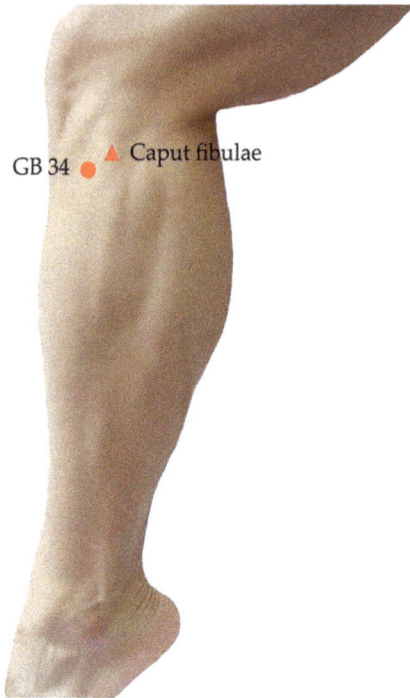

GB 34 ● ▲ Caput fibulae

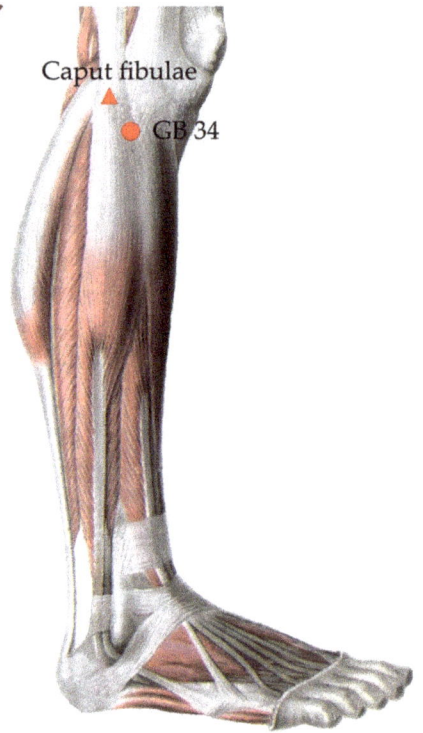

Caput fibulae
▲
● GB 34

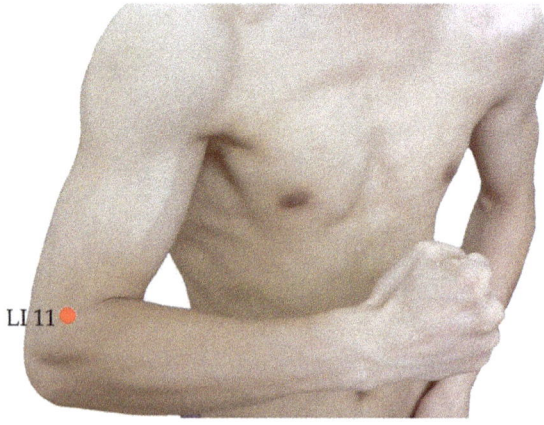

LI 11 ●

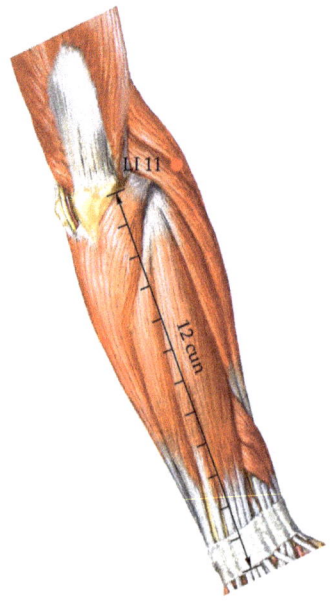

LI 11

12 cun

16. LI-4, LV-3 — Promotes blood flow and alleviates pain, regulates the Qi

Indications	Swelling and pain of the eye, sore throat, irregular menstruation, dysmenorrhea, retention of the placenta, insomnia, distention in the chest and hypochondrium, vomiting, irritability.

LI-4 — HéGǔ

Position	On the dorsum of the hand, between the first and second metacarpal bones, on the radial side of the middle of the second metacarpal bone.
Acupoint Selection Skills	The point is located in the web between the index finger and the thumb when the thumb and index are stretched apart, at the middle point of the first metacarpal bone. Another method is by locating the highest part of the m. adductor pollicis when the thumb and index finger are pressed together.
Regional Anatomy	The needle passes through the subcutaneous tissues, enters the m. interossedorsales (1st), and penetrates the m. adductor pollicis from the medial side of the dorsal venous network and deep palmar artery.
Acupuncture	Insert the needle perpendicularly 0.5~1.0 cun deep and stimulte until there is a sore and numbing sensation in the local area radiating to the fingers.

LV-3 — TàiChōng

Position	On the dorsum of the foot, in the depression between the first and second metatarsal bone.
Acupoint Selection Skills	The point is located in the sitting position with the foot resting on the ground or supine position, on the dorsum of the foot, between the first and second metatarsal bone, in the depression lateral to the tendon of m. extensor pollicis longus.
Regional Anatomy	The needle passes through the subcutaneous tissues and penetrates the m. interos-seidorsales.
Acupuncture	Insert the needle obliquely upwards 0.5~1.0 cun deep and stimulate until there is a sore and numbing sensation in the local area radiating to the sole of the foot.

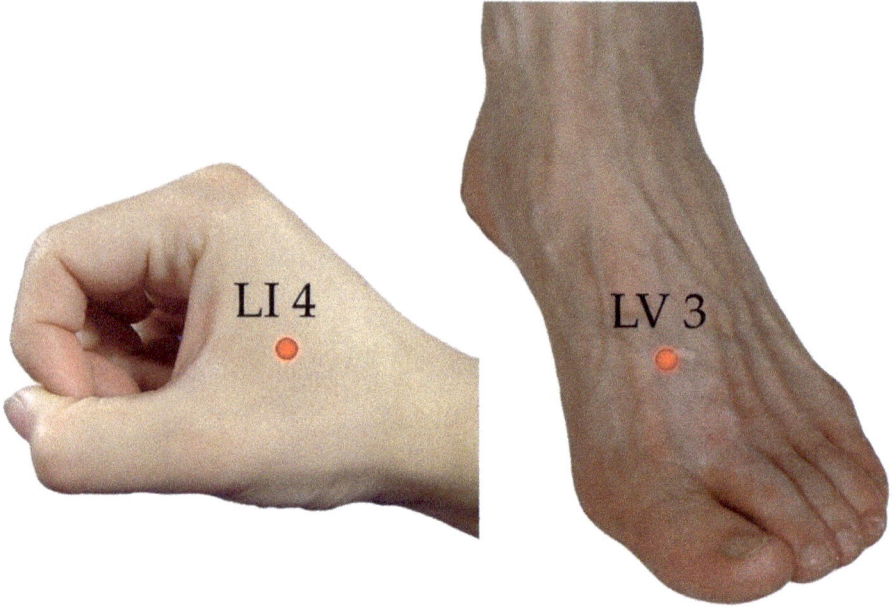

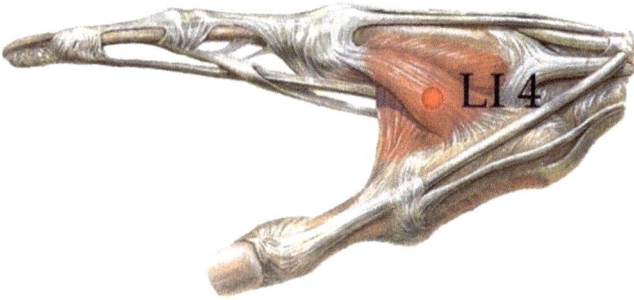

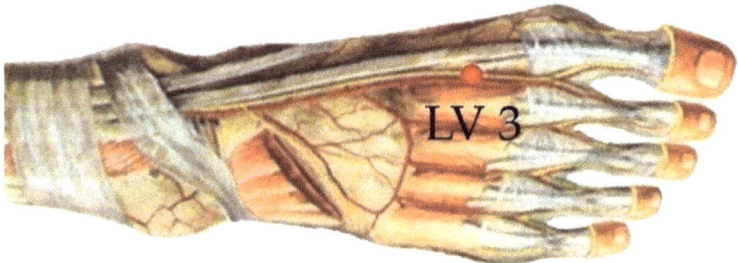

17. BL-40, BL-57 — Relaxes sinews, activates channel and alleviates pain, regulates large intestine

Indications	Joint pain due to stagnation of damp-cold, hemiplegia, hemorrhoids, constipation, pain in the lumbar and lower limbs

BL-40 — WěiZhōng

Position	At the midpoint of the transverse crease of the popliteal fossa.
Acupoint Selection Skills	The point is located in the prone position, in the center of the popliteal fossa, between the tendon of m. biceps femoris and m. semitendinous.
Regional Anatomy	The needle passes through the subcutaneous tissues and penetrates the muscle of pop-liteal fossa.
Acupuncture	Insert the needle perpendicularly 0.5~1.0 cun deep and stimulate until there is a sore, dis-tending and numbing sensation radiating to the calf and foot.

BL-57 — ChéngShān

Position	On the posterior midline of the lower leg, the point is in the depression between m. triceps su-rae and tendon.
Acupoint Selection Skills	The point is located in the prone position, in the depression below the belly of m. gastrocnemius when the lower extremities are flexed with toes extended.
Regional Anatomy	The needle passes through the subcutaneous tissues and penetrates m. tibialis posteri-or.
Acupuncture	Insert the needle obliquely 0.5~1.0 cun deep and stimulate until there is a sore and numb-ing sensation in the local area radiating to the calf and foot.

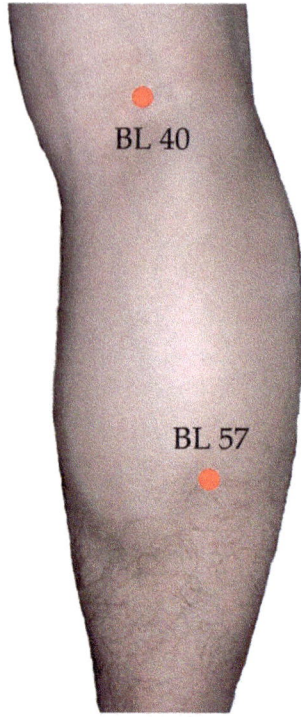

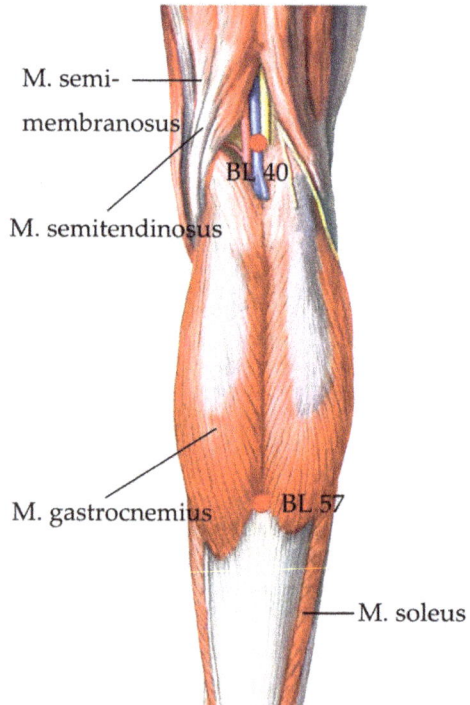

Acupuncture of Acupoint Combination

18. BL-40, PC-3 — Clears heat and cools blood, activates channel and alleviates pain, revives consciousness, clearing away heat and toxic material.

Indications	Erysipelas, boils, furuncle, hyperthermia, stroke, epilepsy, cough and asthma, high blood pressure, acute vomiting and diarrhea.

BL-40 — WěiZhōng

Position	At the midpoint of the transverse crease of the popliteal fossa.
Acupoint Selection Skills	The point is located in the prone position, in the center of the popliteal fossa, between the tendon of m. biceps femoris and m. semitendinous.
Regional Anatomy	The needle passes through the subcutaneous tissues and penetrates the muscle of pop-liteal fossa.
Acupuncture	Insert the needle perpendicularly 0.5~1.0 cun deep and stimulate until there is a sore, dis-tending and numbing sensation radiating to the calf and foot.

PC-3 — QūZé

Position	On the transverse crease of the elbow, on the ulnar side of the tendon of m. biceps brachii.
Acupoint Selection Skills	The point is located when the arm is stretched forward with palm upward and the elbow flexed, on the transverse crease of the elbow.
Regional Anatomy	The needle passes through skin and subcutaneous fascia, pierces the anterior cubital fascia between v. basilica and intermedian cubital vein, reaches the trunk of n. medianus and m. brachialis at the medial side of the brachial artery.
Acupuncture	Insert the needle perpendicularly 0.5~1.0 cun deep and stimulate until there is a numbing and distending sensation in the local area radiating to the the middle finger.

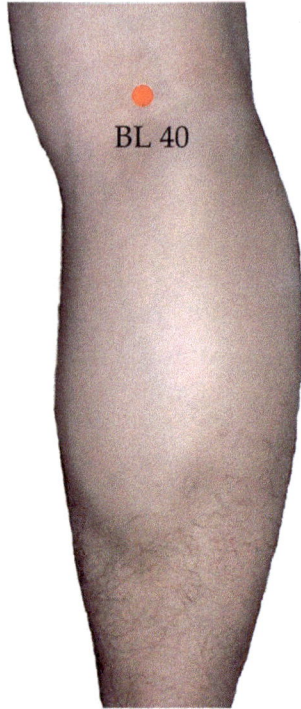
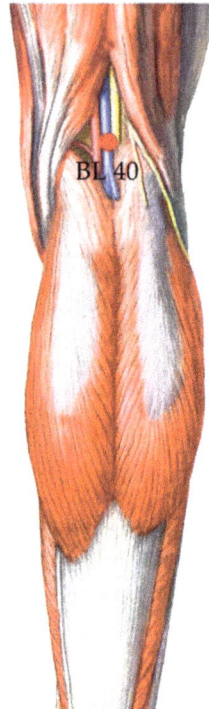

BL 40

BL 40

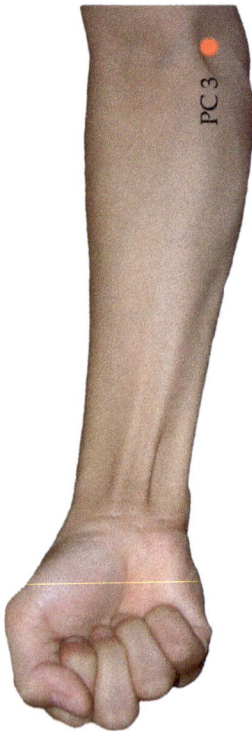
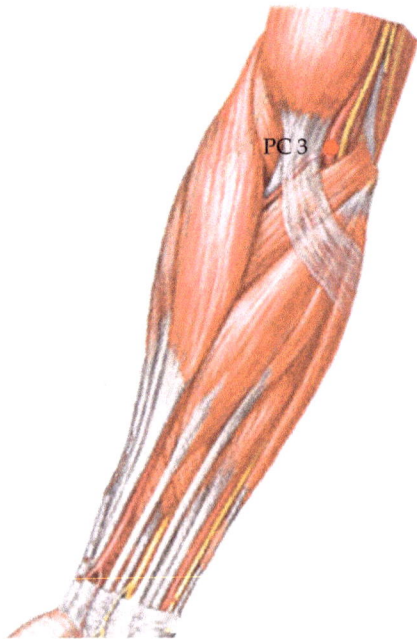

PC 3

PC 3

CHAPTER 5
Systemic Combination Points

1. RN-12, PC-6, ST-36 — Regulates Qi and harmonizes stomach, descends rebellious Qi and alleviates nausea and vomiting

Indications	Diarrhea, vomiting, constipation, abdominal distention, abdominal pain, poor appetite.

RN-12 — ZhōngWǎn

Position	On the upper abdomen, on the anterior midline, 4 cun superior to the umbilicus.
Regional Anatomy	The needle passes through subcutis and penetrates the internal abdominal fascia and subperiotoneal fascia.
Acupuncture	Insert the needle perpendicularly 0.5~1.0 cun deep and stimulate until there is a sore and distending sensation in the local area radiating to the stomach.

PC-6 — NèiGuān

Position	On the palmar aspect of the forearm, 2 cun superior to the transverse crease of the wrist, between the tendon of m.palmaris longus and m. flexor carpi radialis.
Acupoint Selection Skills	The point is located on the forearm with the palm upward and the wrist is slightly flexed, 2 cun superior to the midpoint of the transverse crease of the wrist, on the line connecting PC-3 to PC-7, between the tendon of m.palmaris longus and m. flexor carpi radialis.

Regional Anatomy	The needle passes through the skin and subcutaneous fascia, pierces the deep brachial fascia, reaches m. flexor digitorumsuperficialis between m. palmaris longus and m. flexor carpi radialis, enters m. flexor digitorumprofundus and m. pronator quadratus.
Acupuncture	Insert the needle perpendicularly 0.5~1.5 cun deep and stimulate until there is a sore and numbing sensation in the local area with an electric sensation radiating to the finger tip.

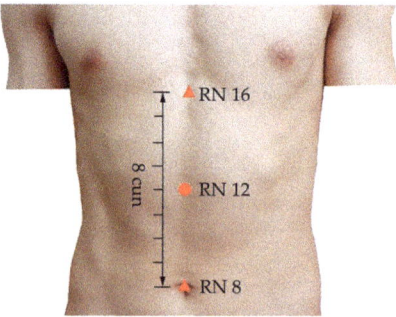

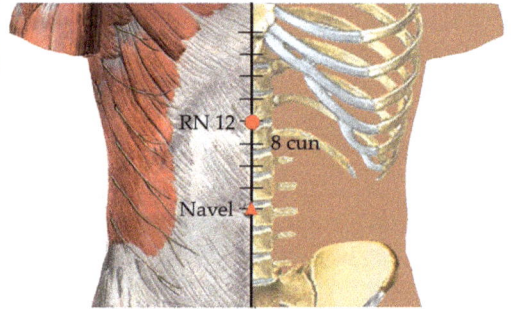

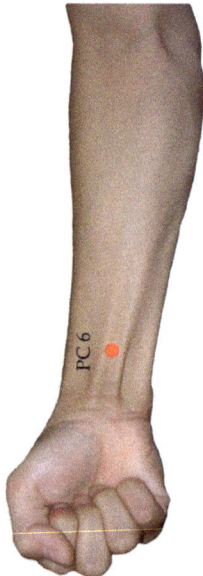

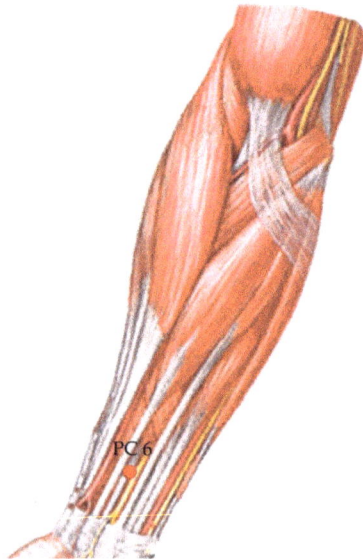

Acupuncture of Acupoint Combination

ST-36 — ZúSānLǐ

Position	On the anterior aspect of the lower leg, 3 cun distal to ST-35, one finger width lateral from the anterior ridge of the tibia.
Acupoint Selection Skills	① The point is located in the sitting position when the knee is bent, 3 cundistal to ST 35, one finger width lateral to the anterior ridge of the tibia. ② The point is located in the sitting position when the knee is bent 1 cun below the outer inferior margin of tibial trochanter.
Regional Anatomy	The needle passes through the subcutaneous tissues and penetrates m. tibialis anterior and m. extensor hallucis longus.
Acupuncture	Insert the needle perpendicularly 0.5~1.5 cun deep and stimulate until there is a sensation radiating to the ankle and dorsum of the foot and toes.

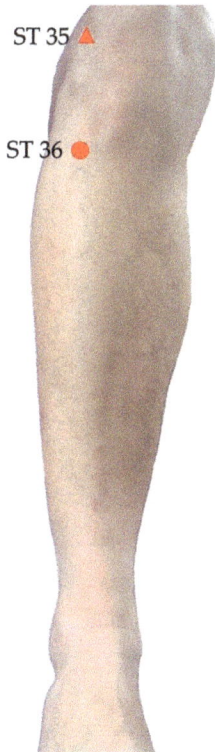

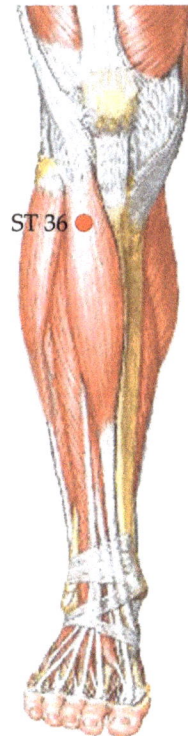

ST 35 ▲

ST 36 ●

ST 36 ●

2. ST-25, ST-37 — Regulates the spleen and stomach, activates the channel and alleviates pain

Indications	Diarrhea, constipation, abdominal distention, acute abdominal disease.

ST-25 — TiānShū

Position	On the abdomen, 2 cun lateral to the umbilicus.
Regional Anatomy	The needle passes through the subcutaneous tissues and penetrates the posterior layer of sheath of m. rectus abdominis and m. rectus abdominis.
Acupuncture	Insert the needle perpendicularly 1.0~1.5 cun deep and stimulate until there is a sore and numbing sensation in the local area radiating to the side of the abdomen.

ST-37 — ShàngJùXū

Position	On the anterior and lateral side of the leg, 6 cun distal to ST-35, one finger width lateral from the anterior ridge of the tibia.
Acupoint Selection Skills	The point is located in the sitting position when the knee is bent or in the supine position, 6 cundistal to ST-35, one finger width lateral to the anterior ridge of the tibia.
Regional Anatomy	The needle passes through the subcutaneous tissues and penetrates m. tibialis anterior and m. extensor hallucis longus.
Acupuncture	Insert the needle perpendicularly 1.0~2.0 cun deep and stimulate until there is a sore and numbing sensation in the local area.

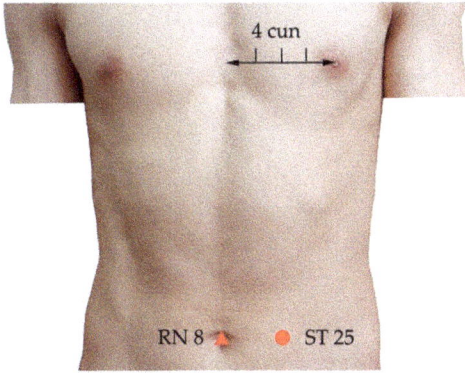

4 cun

RN 8   ST 25

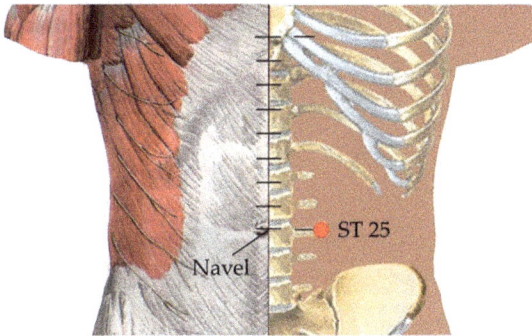

ST 25

Navel

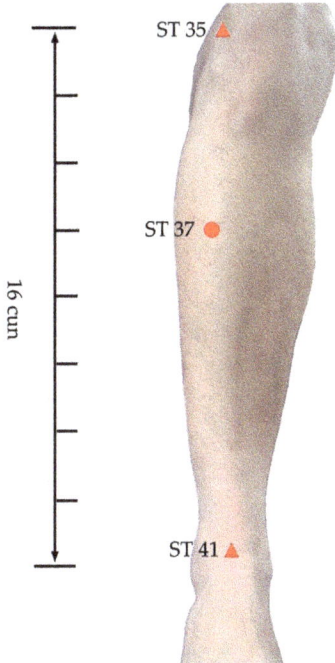

ST 35

ST 37

16 cun

16 cun

ST 41

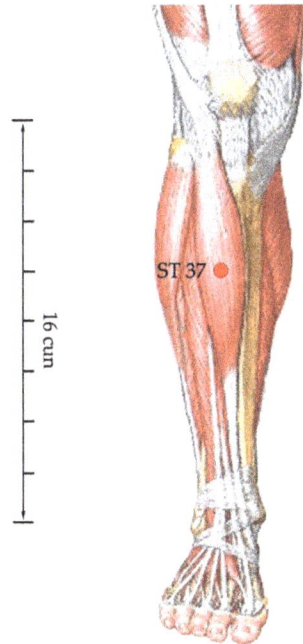

ST 37

3. PC-6, RN-17 — Unbinds the chest and regulates Qi, regulates heart and calms the spirit

Indications	Heart palpitation, irritability and cardiac pain, chest congestion, insomnia, hiccup singultation.

PC-6 — NèiGuān

Position	On the palmar aspect of the forearm, 2 cun superior to the transverse crease of the wrist, between the tendon of m.palmaris longus and m. flexor carpi radialis.
Acupoint Selection Skills	The point is located on the forearm with the palm upward and the wrist is slightly flexed, 2 cun superior to the midpoint of the transverse crease of the wrist, on the line connecting PC-3 to PC-7, between the tendon of m.palmaris longus and m. flexor carpi radialis.
Regional Anatomy	The needle passes through the skin and subcutaneous fascia, pierces the deep brachial fascia, reaches m. flexor digitorumsuperficialis between m. palmaris longus and m. flexor carpi radialis, enters m. flexor digitorumprofundus and m. pronator quadratus.
Acupuncture	Insert the needle perpendicularly 0.5~1.5 cun deep and stimulate until there is a sore and numbing sensation in the local area with an electric sensation radiating to the finger tip.

RN-17 — DànZhōng

Position	On the chest, on the anterior midline, at the level of the fourth intercostal space.
Acupoint Selection Skills	The point is located in the supine position, at the junction of the line connecting the two nipples and the midline of the sternum, at the level with the fourth intercostal space.
Regional Anatomy	The needle passes through subcutis and penetrates the periost of sternal body.

Acupuncture	Insert the needle subcutaneously or obliquely 0.3~0.5 cun deep and stimulate until there is a sore and distending sensation in the local area radiating to the chest.

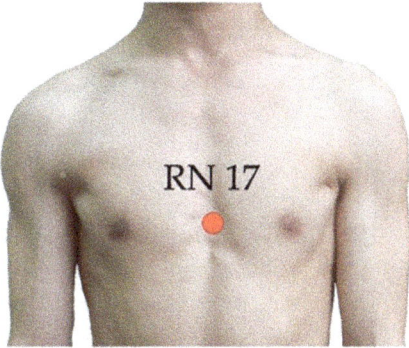

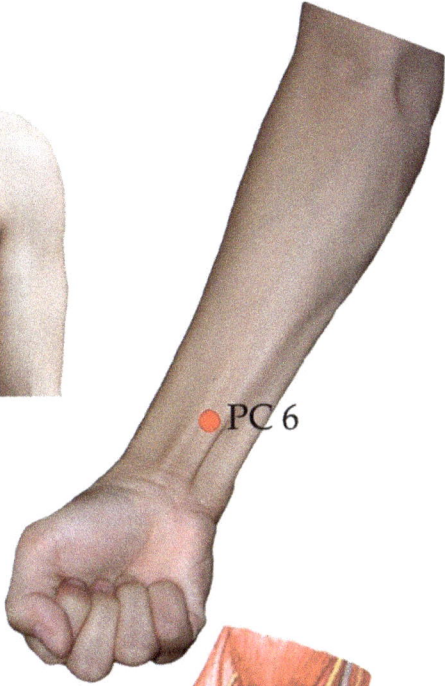

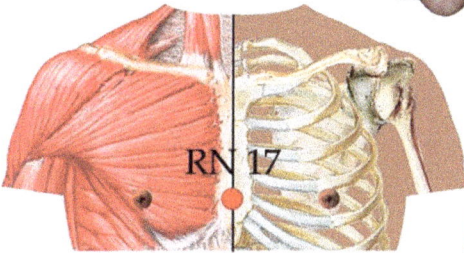

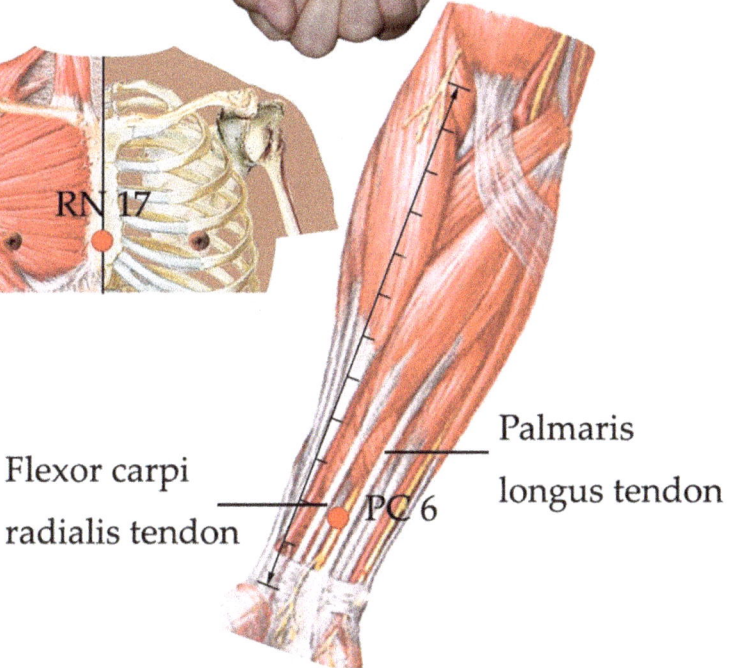

RN 17

PC 6

RN 17

Flexor carpi radialis tendon

PC 6

Palmaris longus tendon

4. LV-3, LV-14 — Unbinds the chest and regulates Qi, clears liver fire and spreads liver Qi

Indications	Pain and distention in the hypochondrium, vomiting, headache, insomnia, irregular, menstruation, amenorrhea, hernia, abdominal pain, irritable.

LV-3 — TàiChōng

Position	On the dorsum of the foot, in the depression between the first and second metatarsal bone.
Acupoint Selection Skills	The point is located in the sitting position with the foot resting on the ground or supine position, on the dorsum of the foot, between the first and second metatarsal bone, in the depression lateral to the tendon of m. extensor pollicis longus.
Regional Anatomy	The needle passes through the subcutaneous tissues and penetrates the m. interosseidorsales.
Acupuncture	Insert the needle obliquely upwards 0.5~1.0 cun deep and stimulate until there is a sore and numbing sensation in the local area radiating to the sole of the foot.

LV-14 — QīMén

Position	On the chest, directly inferior to the nipple, in the sixth intercostal space, 4 cun lateral to the anterior midline.
Acupoint Selection Skills	The point is located in the supine position, two intercostal space inferior to ST-17, in the sixth intercostal space, inferior to the mid-clavicle line. For women, the point is located in the clavicles midline, in the sixth intercostal space.
Regional Anatomy	The needle passes through the subcutaneous tissues and penetrates endothoracic fascia.
Acupuncture	Insert the needle obliquely 0.5~0.8 cun deep and stimulate until there is a sore and numbing sensation in the local area radiating to the back.

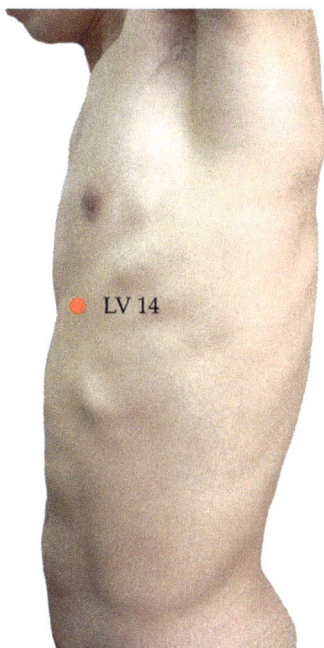

LV 14

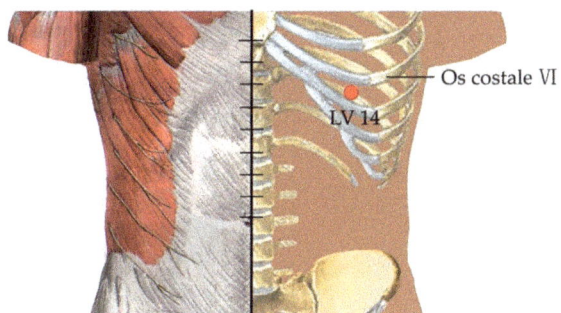

Os costale VI

LV 14

LV 14

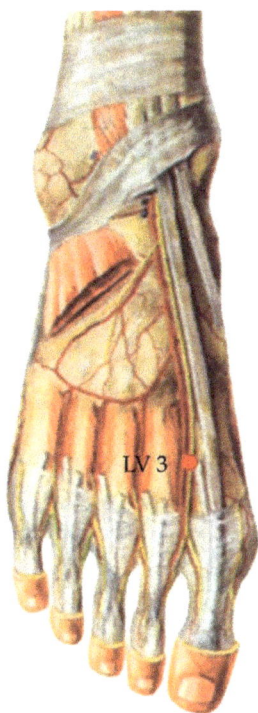

LV 3

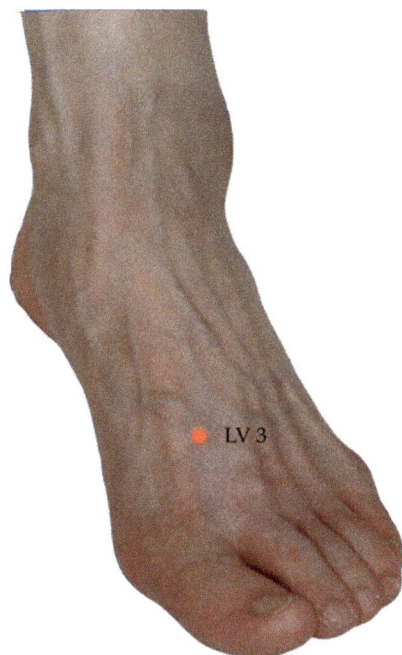

LV 3

5. BL-10, BL-60 — Benefits the head and eyes, activates the channel and activates collaterals

Indications	Headache, dizziness, neck stiffness, epilepsy, nasal obstruction, pain of the lumbosacral region.

BL-10 — TiānZhù

Position	On the neck, in the depression on the lateral border of m. trapezius, superior to the spinous process of the second cervical vertebra.
Acupoint Selection Skills	The point is located in the sitting position with the head bent forward or in the prone position, 1.3 cun lateral to DU-15, lateral to m. trapezius.
Regional Anatomy	The needle passes through the subcutaneous tissues and penetrates m. rectus capitis posterior major.
Acupuncture	Insert the needle perpendicularly or obliquely 0.5~0.8 cun deep and stimulate until there is a sore and numbing sensation in the local area.

BL-60 — KūnLún

Position	On the foot, posterior to the external mallelous, in the depression between the tip of the external mallelous and tendon calcaneus.
Acupoint Selection Skills	The point is located in the sitting position with the foot resting on the ground, in the depression between the tip of the external mallelous and tendon calcaneus.
Regional Anatomy	The needle passes through the subcutaneous tissues and penetrates m. peroneus brevis.
Acupuncture	Insert the needle perpendicularly towards KI-3 0.5~1.5 cun deep and stimulate until there is a sore and numbing sensation in the local area radiating to the heel.

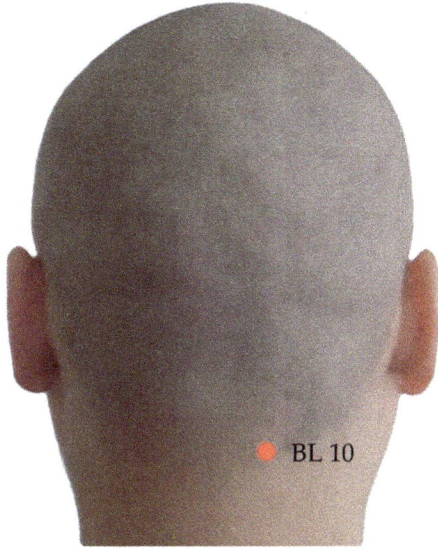

BL 10

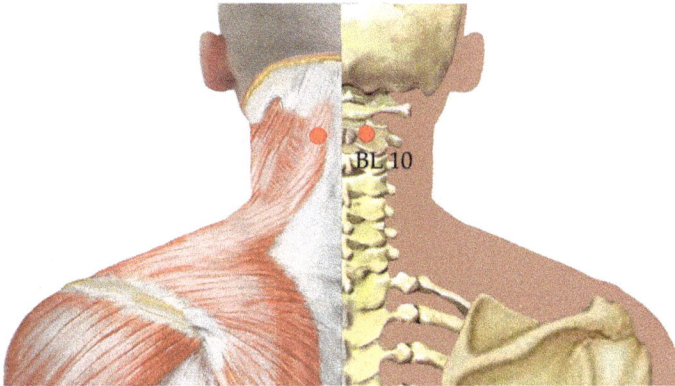

BL 10

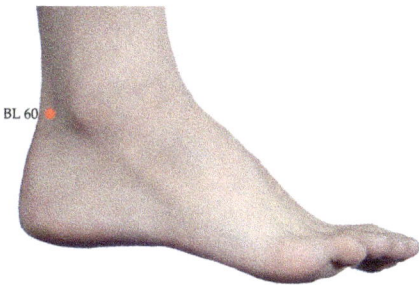

BL 60

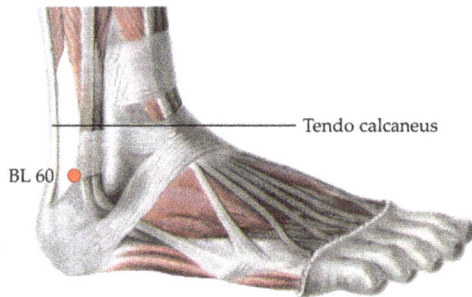

Tendo calcaneus

BL 60

6. BL-23, KI-3 — Nourishes kidney yin and tonifies kidney, tonifies original Qi

Indications	General weakness, tinnitus, enuresis, edema, impotence, amnesia and neurosis, lumbago, amenorrhea, heel pain.

BL-23 — ShènShū

Position	On the lower back, 1.5 cun lateral to the lower border of the spinous process of the second lumbar vertebra.
Acupoint Selection Skills	The point is located in the prone position, at the level with the inferior border of the spinous process of the second lumbar vertebra, 1.5 cun lateral to DU-4 on the opposite side of RN-8.
Regional Anatomy	The needle passes through the subcutaneous tissues and penetrates m. quadratus lumborum and m. psoas major.
Acupuncture	Insert the needle perpendicularly 0.5~1.0 cun deep and stimulate until there is a sore and numbing sensation in the local area radiating to the hip and down the leg.

KI-3 — TàiXī

Position	On the medial aspect of the foot, posterior to the medialmallelous, in the depression between the tip of the medial malleolus and the tendon calcaneus.
Regional Anatomy	The needle passes through the skin and subcutaneous fascia, penetrates the deep crural fascia and runs between the inner ankle and tendo calcaneus.
Acupuncture	Insert the needle perpendicularly toward BL-60 0.5~1.0 cun deep and stimulate until there is a sore and numbing sensation in the local area radiating to the heel.

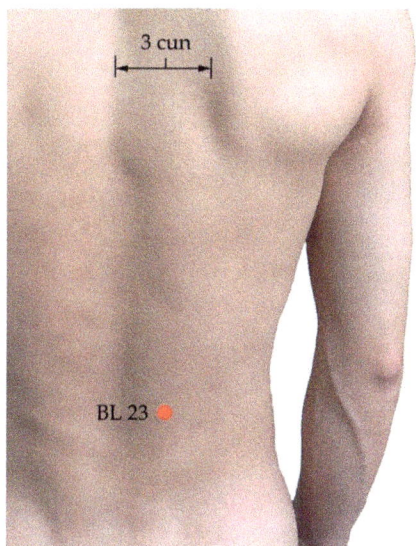

3 cun

BL 23

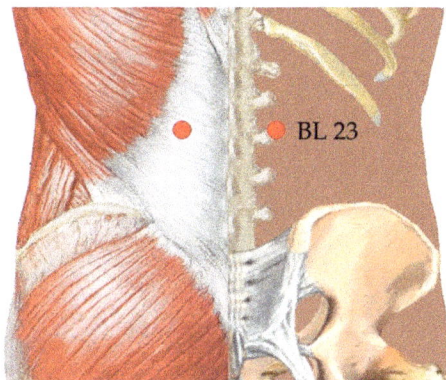

BL 23

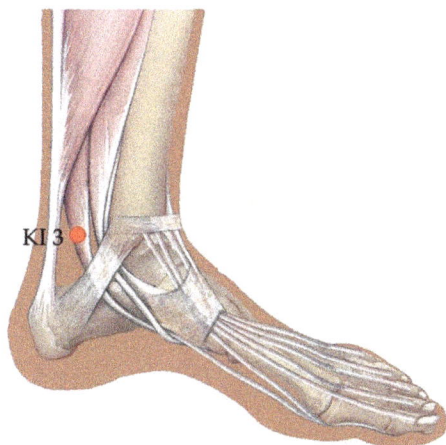

KI 3

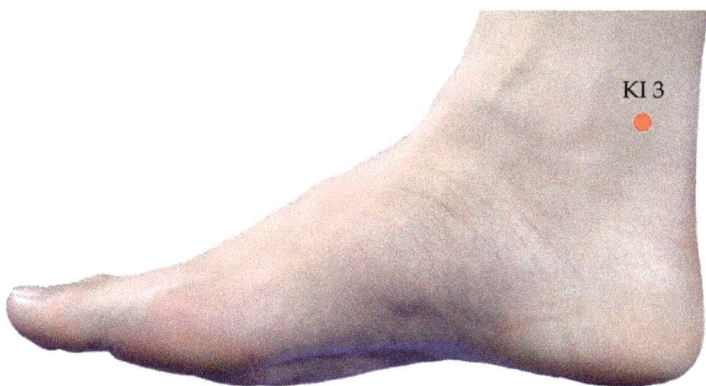

KI 3

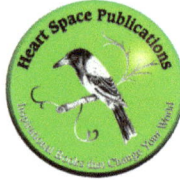

If you derived benefit from this manual,
please see the other three in the series of

Quick Reference Handbooks of Chinese Medicine

Acupuncture – of Acupoint Combinations Quick Lookups

Illustrations Of Special Effective Acupoints for
common Diseases

Human Body Reflex Zone Quick Lookup,
Bilingual anatomical illustration of reflex zones
(English edition)

Quick Investigation On Acupunture Points – Selection of
Professor Yang Jiasan

Go to www.heartspacepublications.com